AF559854

Common Reproductive Problems in Bovines and Canines

— Hand Manual —

www.nipaers.com

Browse, Search, Read & Buy...

Print Books eChapters
eBooks Publishers
Forthcoming Subject Catalogues
New Titles

Online Resources on:

- ✓ Current Affairs
- ✓ Reasoning, Logic & Aptitude
- ✓ Competitive Examinations
- ✓ English Language Lab
- ✓ Writing & Pronunciation Tools
- ✓ Personality Development
- ✓ Online Programmes for Professionals
- ✓ Interview Preparation

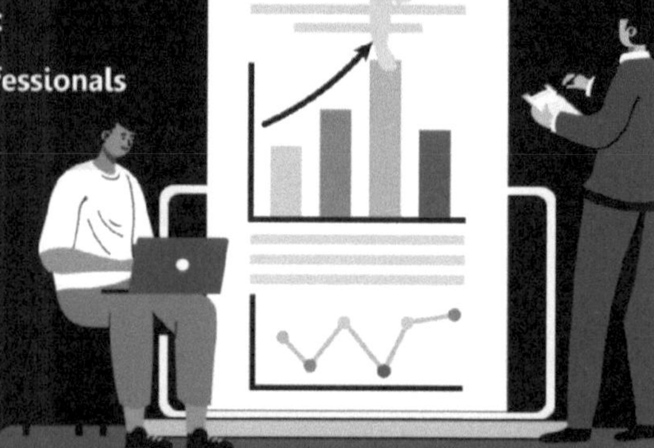

Pay Using

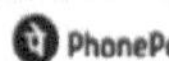

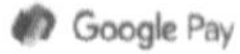

paytm
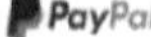

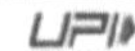

CC Avenue

Common Reproductive Problems in Bovines and Canines
— Hand Manual —

Dr Harendra Kumar
B.Sc, B.V.Sc & A.H., M.V.Sc, Ph.D.
Principal Scientist
Division of Animal Reproduction

Dr S. Nandi
B.V.Sc & A.H., M.V.Sc, Ph.D.
Senior Scientist
Centre for Animal Disease Research and Diagnosis

Dr R.B. Rai
B.V.Sc & A.H., M.V.Sc, Ph.D.
Principal Scientist
Division of Veterinary Pathology

INDIAN VETERINARY RESEARCH INSTITUTE
IZATNAGAR, UTTAR PRADESH (INDIA)

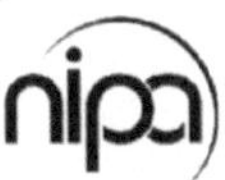

New India Publishing Agency
Pitam Pura, New Delhi-110 088

Published by
Sumit Pal Jain *for*

New India Publishing Agency
101, Vikas Surya Plaza, CU Block, L.S.C. Mkt.,
Pitam Pura, New Delhi-110 088, (India)
Ph.: 011-27341616, Fax: 011-27341717, Mob.: 09717133558
E-mail: newindiapublishingagency@gmail.com
Web: www.bookfactoryindia.com

© Authors: **2011**

All rights reserved, no part of this publication may be reproduced, stored in a retrieval system or transmitted in any form or by any means, electronic, mechanical, photocopying, recording or otherwise without the prior written permission of the publisher/editor.

This book contains information obtained from authentic and highly regarded sources. Reasonable efforts have been made to publish reliable data and information, but the authors/editor(s)/contributors and publisher cannot assume responsibility for the validity of all materials or the consequences of their use. The authors/editor(s)/contributors and publisher have attempted to trace and acknowledge the copyright holders of all material reproduced in this publication and apologize to copyright holders if permission and acknowledgements to publish in this form have not been given. If any copyright material has not been acknowledged please write and let us know so we may rectify it.

ISBN : 978-93-95763-90-5

Composed and Designed by NIPA

Dedicated
to our
Beloved Parents

Preface

The livestock sector in India is experiencing fast growth. Livestock resources across regions and species have therefore to be utilized optimally to achieve the goals of efficiency, equity, nutritional security and sustainability. Consumption of livestock products has been increasing over the last 20 years. Sustained economic growth and attendant increase in per capita income are expected to further boost demand of livestock products substantially. Demand for milk and meat is estimated to be 147 and 14 million tonnes, respectively, in 2020. Changing consumption pattern and increasing needs of livestock products would demand use of new scientific technologies to achieve goal of increased animal production efficiency. It is obvious that reproduction comes before production and thus, it becomes essential to update the practical knowledge for achieving optimum fertility from our dairy animals.

This new ***"Common Reproductive Problems in Bovines and Canines - Hand Manual"*** deals with nearly all aspects of reproductive disorders in cows, buffaloes & bitches under a single cover. We do believe that this, compilation of knowledge/information, will benefit to our veterinary clinicians, field workers as well as students. This has been written to fulfill the gap and aimed to provide desired knowledge as well as putting the management of reproductive health control in dairy and pet animals, in the hands of Veterinarians.

My humble researches in the field of Veterinary Gynaecology and Obstetrics specially on the diagnosis and therapeutic management of all kind of reproductive disorders in animals have convinced me to put my research findings and experiences obtained through studies at organized farms and subsequently by field trials together experiences gained during handling the clinical cases at IVRI polyclinic as well as at farmer's door, in the form of a "Hand Manual" to the hands of field Veterinarians. I am sure that this will give them a detailed understanding of the subjects in concise and systemic manner. I hope that with the help of this manual they should be in a position to follow the important therapeutics methods in cows, buffalos as well as in bitches to improve their reproductive efficiency.

Dr. Harendra Kumar
Dr. Sukdeb Nandi
Dr. R.B. Rai

Contents

Bovines

CHAPTER 1

CLINICAL GUIDANCE FOR GYNAECOLOGICAL EXAMINATION OF BOVINES

RECTAL EXAMINATION

- It provides practically all the information required.
- It is the simplest, accurate and reliable method with no cost involved.

Things Required

- A full arm rubber sleeve with attached glove or disposable plastic glove.
- A rubber or plastic apron.
- Non-irritant soap or lubricant.

Restraining of The Animal

- By putting in a trevis (commonly available) or chute.

- If the trevis is not available restrain the cow/ buffalo against a tree.

Entry into Rectum

- Enter the fingers and the hand in the form of a cone after proper lubrication.
- Enter beyond the pelvic brim and bring back the hand along with a fold of rectum.
- If necessary remove the dung.
- If there is any peristaltic wave, remove the hand in heifers and small animals and in others stop examining and allow it to pass over.
- If the rectum is ballooned with air, stimulate peristalsis by massaging of the rectal wall prior to the anus and hooking the fingers cranially in the contraction ring and pulling it backwards.
- Be careful, gentle to the animal.
- If there is bleeding, stop examination.

Common Causes of Rectal Trauma

- Too much force.
- Too long a period of examination.
- Manipulations with distended air.
- Manipulations during peristaltic wave.
- Long finger nails.

Orientation and Landmarks

Rectal examination depends on the tactile sense.

- It requires landmarks for general orientation and recognition of organs.
- The pelvic inlet in general and the pelvic brim in particular provide excellent landmarks for orientation during rectal examination.
- Failure to identify the uterus positively is one of the most frequent reasons for diagnostic errors.
- Hence a systematic approach to identify and examine the uterus is imperative.
- The cervix because of its distinct characteristics and relatively constant position provides an useful landmark.

LOCATION AND EXAMINATION OF THE CERVIX

- Location of cervix represents the first step.
- The arm is inserted far enough to palpate the pelvic inlet.
- The hand with the fingers slightly bent is swept along one of the walls of the pelvic cavity down to the floor and over to the other side.
- If the cervix is not located in the first sweep, the process is repeated at different depths until is found.
- The cervix is recognized as a **firm, cylindrical** and somewhat **nodular** structure lying on the **midline** of the pelvic floor.

- In nonpregnant cows the cervix is mostly located in the middle of pelvic cavity with the whole uterus within the pelvic cavity.
- In nonpregnant buffalo cows it is more posterior in location.
- In exotic and older animals and in pregnant animals the cervix may be located over the pelvic brim.

Size

- Varies with age, stage of reproductive cycle and the presence or absence of abnormalities.
- Length is about 7.5 to 10 cm and width is about 2.0 to 6.0 cm.
- Slightly tapers off towards the internal os.
- Size increases with age, parity and disease status.
- Enlargement is more prominent in the posterior end.
- In pregnant cow, it does not enlarge before relaxation.
- Edema becomes prominent early in the first stage of labour.
- Involution proceeds at a slower rate than other segments of the uterus so that it still might be enlarged at the time when the involution of uterine horns is completed. This is also observed after abortion.

Form

- Distinct form.
- Slight lobulation caused by the presence of 3 or 4 annular rings.
- Semiconical form does not change with size.
- Enlargement and distortion of form of the external os seen in older cows.

Common Abnormalities

- Cervicitis - causes local constrictions and consistency changes.
- Abscesses - directly or indirectly involving the cervix are ordinarily very hard and irregular in form.

Position or Location

- In nonpregnant animals mostly within pelvic cavity.
- A full bladder may displace it side ways.
- In older animals and in certain exotic breeds may be at pelvic brim or abdomen
- Early pregnancy (upto 90 days) - within pelvic cavity
- Late pregnancy - over pelvic brim or abdominal.

Mobility

- The cervix is freely mobile in nonpregnant and early pregnant animals up to 60-70 days.

- It is immobile and fixed by the weight of the uterus in late pregnancy and also by the involuting uterus upto 10-14 days postpartum.
- Cervix may also be fixed in pathological conditions like pyometra, mucometra, hydrometra, tumour or adhesions.

EXAMINATION OF THE UTERUS

After location and examination of cervix the uterus or the uterine horns which are the most important parts of the uterus as far as examination is concerned, have to be examined. An experienced examiner when he dips his palm to the pelvic floor comes in contact with uterus with its bifurcation straight away in nonpregnant and early pregnant animals.

Body of The Uterus

- It is immediately anterior to the cervix and is very short approximately 2 to 3 cm.
- The wall is thinner than the other parts of uterus.

Horns of Tthe Uterus

- Bovine uterus is bicornual.
- True bifurcation is at the site of junction with the body of the uterus.
- False bifurcation is further forward at the site where both the horns are connected by two ligamentous sheets - dorsal and ventral intercornual ligaments, of which the ventral ligament is stronger.
- The horns are tubular and twisted like ram's horns.

- The diameter tapers off towards the ovarian end.
- The length of the horns varies from 25 to 40 cm.
- The diameter or width of the horn is much more important in clinical examination than the length and is about 1.5 to 3 cm.
- Slight asymmetry of the width of the horns is present in all but virgin animals.
- The thick wall consists practically entirely of the myometrium and the lumen is not palpable in normal nonpregnant animals.

Broad Ligaments

- The uterus including the cervix and a short segment of the anterior part of the vagina are suspended by the two broad ligaments.
- The ligamentous sheets are covered on both sides by peritoneum carrying blood and lymph vessels and nerves to the internal genital organs.
- They are attached to the uterus at the concave surface or lesser curvature of the horns and laterally to the body and cervix.
- They extend laterally and dorsally to the body wall in the dorso lateral quadrant.
- The anterior edge is oval and forms the utero ovarian ligament and mesovarium.
- The ovaries are suspended approximately 5 cm lateral to the ovarian end of uterine horn.

Retraction of The Uterus

- It is important for complete examination of the uterus especially in larger animals.
- The important thing is to place the uterus in a position where everything can be felt rather than try to trace the horn in their original position.
- Especially in buffaloes it is very difficult to trace the full length the of horns without retraction or rolling up.

Indirect Method of Retraction

Most reliable and is successful in most of the animals.

- After the cervix is located and found to be freely movable, it is pulled back as far as possible by placing the fingers beneath and the thumb on its top.
- The cervix is tilted so that its long axis is perpendicular and the uterus comes closer.
- Then the thumb is also moved underneath the body of the uterus.
- Afterwards the anterior edge of the broad ligament is grasped by turning the hand outward, lowering the bent fingers and hooking the broad ligament.
- By this method the broad ligament is grasped at the angle between the ovarian end of the horn and the ovary.

- The bent fingers are then slide medially and the horn is gathered up in the palm.
- This is possible also with pregnant horn of animals upto 70 days pregnant.
- The horn is brought backward and the fingers are slid further medially until a good hold on the ventral intercornual ligament is obtained.
- The false bifurcation is then brought back and the horns are deflected or rolled back.
- This places the horns of the uterus in the posterior part of the pelvic cavity and the retraction is completed.

Retraction by Direct Method

- The cervix is grasped and pulled back as far as possible.
- The groove between both horns is then followed forward until the anterior edge of the dorsal intercornual ligament is palpated.
- Slight traction is exerted on this ligament to bring the ventral ligament which is then grasped and the retraction is completed as described above.

Examination of The Uterine Horns

- Performed by tracking and palpating entire length of the individual horns starting from the base upto the ovarian end with the thumb on one side and the other fingers on another side of the horn.

- The first question to be answered is whether or not the animal is pregnant.
- The diagnosis that an animal is not pregnant should never be made unless both horns of the uterus have been thoroughly examined in their entire length.

EXAMINATION OF THE OVARIES

Ovaries should be routinely examined in all animals found to be nonpregnant. Palpation of ovaries is contraindicated in pregnant animals except in very early pregnancy because it gives no useful information and if the corpus luteum is damaged pregnancy will be disrupted.

Anatomy

- Bovine ovaries are almond or oval shaped when they do not contain any large functional structures.
- Length from pole is about 1.5 to 2.5 cm. Width from surface to surface is 1.0 to 2.0 cm. Height from attached to free border is 1.5 to 2.0 cm.
- Ovaries are large in older animals and smaller in heifers.
- Ovarian stroma, with the exception of functional corpora lutea and follicles is firm and nodular.

Palpation of Ovaries

- The ovaries are usually located on the pelvic floor about 3 cm lateral to the cervix and usually about 3 cm cranial to internal os.
- The ovaries may also be traced from the tip of the uterine horns slightly posterior and lateral to them.

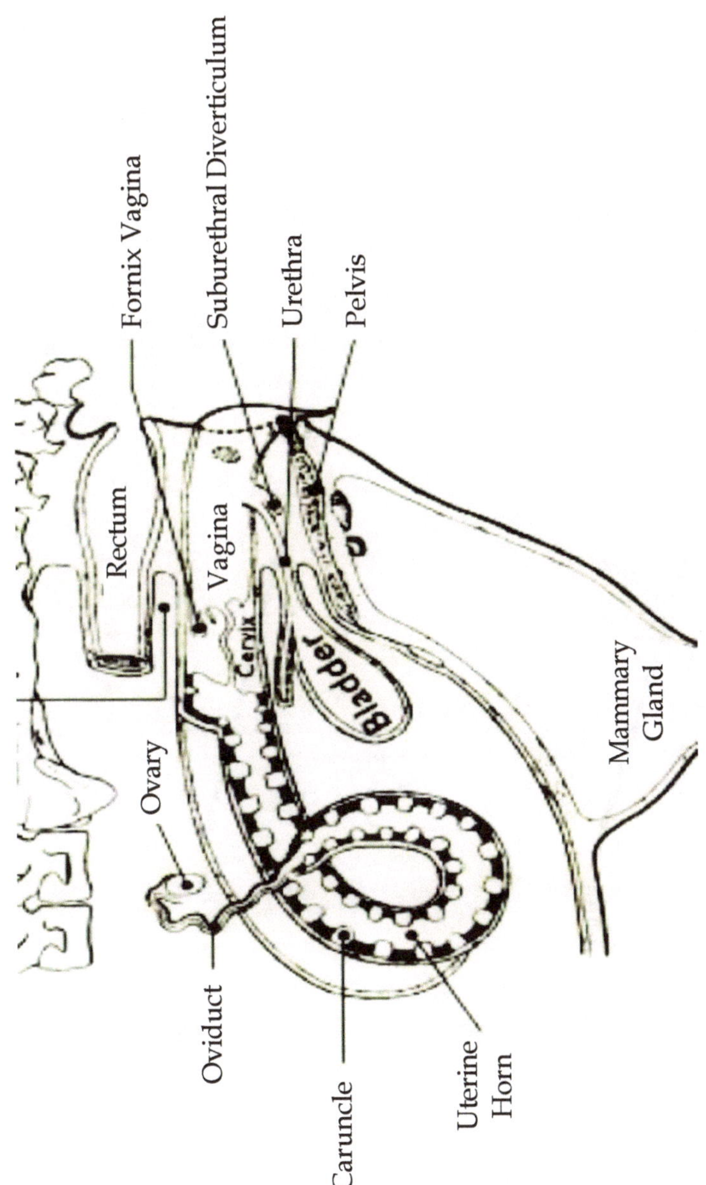

Plate - 1 : Genital Organs of a Cow

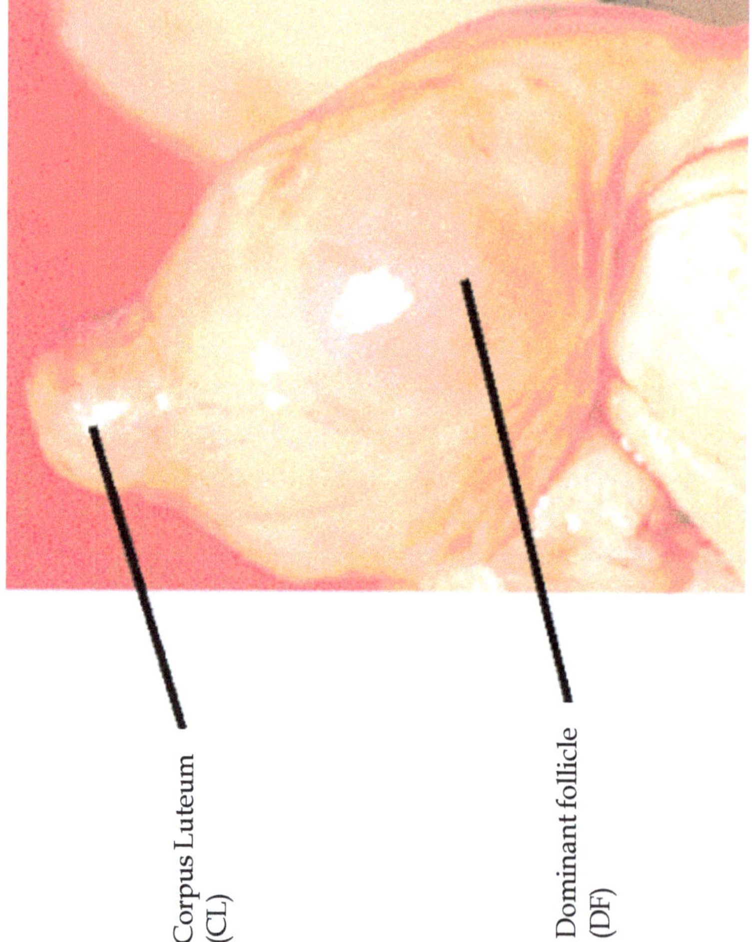

Plate - 2 : Corpus Luteum in the Ovary of a Cow

- Another method of locating the ovary is by hooking the anterior border of the broad ligament with bent fingers and tracing it along its anterior border.
- Once the ovary is located it is lifted up and held between the two middle fingers and the surface is palpated with the thumb.

EXAMINATION OF THE OVIDUCTS AND THE OVARIAN BURSA

Because of the functional significance of the oviducts, detection of abnormalities is extremely important. Many times abnormalities leading to functional disturbance might not be detectable by rectal palpation.

Anatomy

- An oviduct is a narrow coiled tube 20-25 cm long.
- The width is uniform about 2 mm except the proximal 5 to 8 cms where the oviduct widens gradually forming the funnel or the infundibulum, the opening of which is located in opposition to the anterior pole of the ovary.
- The consistency is very hard and cord like except the infundibulum.
- It is suspended in a separate ligamentous sheet, the mesosalpinx which is found ventral to the mesovarium.
- Mesosalpinx and mesovarium form a pocket, the ovarian bursa which is approximately 4 to 6 cm deep and twice as wide.

Examination

- Palpation of the ovarian bursa involves locating the ovary and extending the fingers in the direction cranial, ventral and lateral to the ovary into the bursa.
- Spreading of fingers exposes the bursa which is hooked onto the thumb and lifted up.
- The oviduct is recognized as a coiled cordlike structure that might be followed to the infundibulum laterally and to the uterine horn medially.
- In normal animals the ovarian bursa should be free from adhesions.
- The clinically detectable abnormalities include those directly involving the oviduct and those which affect the mesosalpinx and other surrounding structures. Some of the them are:
  - Segmental aplasia
  - Hydrosalpinx
  - Perisalpingitis and ovarobursal adhesions

❑❑❑

CHAPTER 2

Pregnancy Diagnosis in Cattle & Buffaloes

- Accurate early diagnosis of pregnancy is essential for successful breeding programme.
- Ability is required for successful practice.
- Skill is to be developed to indicate the duration within weeks in early and months in late pregnancy.

External Indications

- Cessation of estrum - under field conditions hardly an useful information.
- Increase in abdominal size - not reliable.

- Enlargement and edema of udder - it begins around 5th month in heifers while in older cows it appears in last month of pregnancy.
- Relaxation of pelvic ligaments and edema and relaxation of vulva visible in last weeks.

Internal Indications on Rectal Examination

Pregnancy diagnosis is based on the following:

1. Presence of the amniotic vesicle.
2. Increase in size of the uterus - dissimilarity.
3. Fluid feeling and thinning of the uterus.
4. Slipping of the fetal membranes.
5. Feel of the fetus and its bump.
6. Feel of the cotyledons.
7. Enlargement of the middle uterine artery.
8. Presence of CL.

   - Above signs are present in all pregnancies.
   - However, certain signs alone are not enough to declare an animal as pregnant.

Positive Signs of Pregnancy are:

- Feeling of Amniotic vesicle
- Feeling of Fetal membranes slip
- Palpation of Fetus/Fetal bump
- Feeling of Cotyledons

"Without confirming anyone of these positive signs no cow should be declared pregnant"

Uterine Changes During Pregnancy

- The gravid horn and to a lesser extent the nongravid horn increase in size because of the growing fetus and fetal fluid - leading to an enlargement and dissimilarity in size between the horns.
- The increase in size leads to thinning of the uterine wall giving a characteristic fluid, watery "alive" feeling.
- From 40-90 days the uterus feels somewhat like a thick rubber balloon nearly filled with water.
- The uterus remains mostly in the pelvic cavity upto 3 months afterwards descends into the abdominal cavity.

Amniotic Vesicle

- Palpable in the free part of the uterine horn from about 30 days because of its tense nature.
- Up to about 40 days it remains spherical after which it becomes oval.
- After 50-55 days it loses it tenseness and is not palpable.

Method of Examination

- The bifurcation of the uterine horns is located.

- The horns are uncoiled and gently palpated along their entire length between the thumb and middle two fingers
- The amniotic sac can be felt as a distinct round or oval turgid object (like a soft shelled hen's egg) slipping between the fingers.
- The sac should not be compressed directly but gently pushed backwards and forwards.
- Usually be located in the pregnant horn in the vicinity of greatest fluid enlargement and thinning of uterine walls.

Fetal Membrane Slip

- Best performed between 35 and 90 days.

Method of Examination

- Identify the bifurcation of uterine horns.
- Pick up and pinch or compress the enlarged gravid horn between the thumb and either the index or middle finger just cranial to the bifurcation.
- Allow the structures to slip and identify the slipping of the fetal membrance first and then the uterine wall (Double slipping).
- In very early pregnancy - it is recommended to grasp the entire horn and let it slip on the ventral aspect so that the thicker connective tissue band can be easily recognized.

- After 70 days of gestation it is often easier to slip in the nongravid horn.

Fetus

- Palpation of the fetus before 75 days is not possible because of the smaller size and tenseness of the amniotic sac.
- Rocking of the flat hand over the enlarged uterus sets the fetal fluids in motion and results in rebounce of the fetus against the hand (fetal bump). Upto 4-5 months the fetal bump can be easily made.
- In late gestation after 8 months fetal parts (not bump) are easily palpable.

Placentomes

- Become recognizable by rectal palpation at about 80-90 days.
- First felt in the mid line by pressing down the uterine body and the base of horns.
- In early stages it is difficult to identify them as distinct individual structures.
- The uterus feels as if it has an irregular corrugated surface and feels like a sack full of small potatoes.
- Once the uterus sunk into the abdomen between 5 and 7 months it is frequently impossible to palpate them.

Hypertrophy and Fremitus of the Middle Uterine Arteries

- In nongravid an early pregnancy - impossible to identify.
- The artery runs is the broad ligament along a tortuous course passing downwards and forwards over the pelvic brim.
- Inexperienced persons sometime confuse it with iliac and obturator arteries which are highly fastened.
- Middle uterine artery is very mobile and can be encircled with the thumb and finger.
- The characteristic hypertrophy and "whirring" (feels like, water surging intermittently through a thin rubber house) is noted in pregnant cows.

PALPATION AT DIFFERENT STAGES

35-40 days

- Requires more skill.
- Easily detectable in heifers and difficult in older cows.
- Uterus in the pelvic cavity.
- Slight enlargement on the free part of one horn with fluid feeling.
- Detectable dorsal bulging.
- Amniotic sac about the size of the yolk of a hen's egg.
- CL ipsilateral to the horn containing amnion.

45-50 days

- Uterus in the pelvic cavity
- Difference in size of pregnant and nonpregnant horn.
- Dorsal bulging more pronounced.
- Amnion about the size of hen's egg (soft shelled egg).
- Membrane slip.

60 days

- Uterus in the pelvic cavity.
- Uterus feels like a narrow ballon filled with water.
- Dissimilarity of horns.
- Membranes slip in both horns.
- Amnion not detectable
- Diameter of the gravid horn is about 6-9 cm.

90 days

- The uterus may be still in the pelvic cavity or over the pelvic brim.
- Uterus about the size of a football bladder.
- Dissimilarity of horns.
- Fetal bump easily palpable.
- Diameter of the gravid horn is about 10-13 cm.
- Cotyledons palpable.
- Fremitus detected.

120 days

- The uterus descends into the abdomen.
- Uterine contour is still palpable.
- Fetus can be palpated.
- Small placentomes can be identified.
- Diameter of the gravid horn is about 12.5-18 cm.
- Fremitus quite distinct.

150 days

- Uterus in the abdominal cavity.
- The cervix over the pelvic brim.
- Distinct crowded Placentomes about the size of ovaries palpable.
- Fetus may or may not be palpable.

170-230 days

- Cervix at the brim of the pelvis.
- Tight cord like folds of uterus running deep into the abdomen from the cervix.
- Uterus difficult to palpate.
- Placentomes and fetus also difficult to palpate.

230-280 days

- The fetus extends back towards the pelvic cavity.
- The head and front feet palpable.
- Movement of fetus and fetal reflex can be detected.

DIFFERENTIAL DIAGNOSIS

Bladder

- A beginner is likely to mistake a filled bladder for gravid uterus.
- Identify the cervix first.
- Trace from the cervix to check whether the enlarged mass is in continuation with the cervix.
- If it is so then indeed the uterus.
- If not trace for the uterus - may be deflected side ways by the bladder.

Rumen

- Rumen feels like a doughy, flaccid mass whereas the gravid uterus gives a live fluid feeling.
- Tracing from the cervix would reveal the uterus.

Pyometra

Pregnancy	Pyometra
Dissimilar horns	Similar horns except in cows where the uterine involution is not complete.
Uterine wall thin	Uterine wall thick
Live fluid feeling	A thick fluid with no resilience.
Double slipping, fetus, Placentomes palpable Depending on the stage of pregnancy	No such positive signs of pregnancy

Metritis

- Thick uterine wall with no fluid feeling.
- Foul smelling discharge in metritis easily identifiable.

Mummified Fetus

Normal Pregnancy	Mummified fetus
Presence of fetal fluids, Placentomes and live fetus	Absence of fluid & Placentomes and the uterus tightly contracted over a semisolid to solid fetal mass
Fremitus Present	Mostly absent

SUMMARY OF RECOMMENDATIONS

- Pregnancy examination should always represent the first step of genital examination.
- No animal should be treated unless the operator is positive that the animal is not pregnant.
- No animal should be pronounced nonpregnant unless both the horns of the uterus have been palpated carefully throughout their entire length.
- A diagnosis of pregnancy should never be made unless the positive signs of pregnancy have been detected and recognized beyond doubt.
- Breeding history should only serve as supplementary information.

- There are certain times, certain animals and certain stages of pregnancy when the positive diagnosis is impossible even for an experienced operator. The "Golden Rule" advises one to admit the inability or doubtfulness and to recommend the re-examination of animal.

❑❑❑

CHAPTER 3

Common Reproductive Problems in Cattle and Buffalo

Case-1

TRUE ANESTRUS IN A HEIFER OR POST PARTUM COW / BUFFALO

- The animal has both ovaries small and inactive
- No palpable structures in the ovaries
- Animal does not exhibiting estrus signs

Causes

- A low plane of nutrition (Under nutrition)- most common cause ie; lack of energy (carbohydrates) and protein, deficiency of minerals like Ca, P, Fe, Cu, Co, Zn, I & Mn and Vitamins A and E or both.

- High milk yield may cause negative energy balance.
- Chronic debilitating diseases – like TB, JD etc. and senility.
- Seasonal and environmental influence.
- Closely confined dark sheds, lack of exercise combined with nutritive factors.
- Suckling - prolactin reduces the ovarian sensitivity.
- These all factors results in insufficient release of gonadotrophins from the anterior pituitary or failure of the ovaries to respond.

Diagnosis

(i) By Rectal Palpation-

- Small & smooth ovaries
- In Buffaloes – spindle like ovaries
- Should be confirmed by repeated examinations at 10 days interval.
- Note abnormal feeding habits like pica etc.

(ii) By Physical Examination-

- Body condition score : e g; < 3

The animal is weak; ribs are clearly visible, less fat in tail (particularly in buffaloes).

Treatment (Rx)

- Improve the nutrition 1st.
- Extra feeding of concentrate mixture or grains like Maize, Gram etc alongwith green fodders like Berseem, Lucern or Cowpea etc.
- Supplement essential minerals for atleast 4 weeks.
- Feed the animal specially chelated mineral mixture.

Area specific mineral mixture-which contains important minerals deficit in that particular area. Or IVRI -Formulation.

- Erradication of all internal and external parasitism by providing broad spectrum anthelmintic drugs.
- Eliminations of all possible stressful factors.
- Attention should be given to improve the general body condition score of the animal.
- Lugol's tampooning at cervix twice a week alongwith ovarian massage for three weeks.
- Feeding of some herbal inducers like: Prajana/ Sajani cap., alongwith cofecu Tab.
- Watch the animal for onset of heat.

❑❑❑

Case-2

ANESTRUS IN A HEIFER OR POST PARTUM COW / BUFFALO

- The ovaries may be medium size & sub active
- Animal does not appear into estrus

Causes

- Deficiency of protein or particular minerals like Ca or P (imbalanced feeding)
- High lactating cows/buffaloes
- Poor management
- Miscellaneous / indirect causes like season or stress etc.

Diagnosis

By History & Rectal examination

- Medium size ovaries
- May be confirmed by repeated gynaecological examination

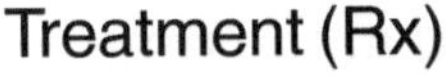

- Provide balanced ration ie; increase the quantity of concentrates to the animal including all macro & micro elements.
- Attention should also be given to improve the general body condition score of the animal.
- Deworming by administration of broad spectrum anthelmintics.
- Ist supplementation of mineral mixture in feed/ ration for 3 to 4 weeks.
- Then administration of progesterone therapy for 5 days (250 mg injection of Proluton or Duraprogen or Uniprogestin daily I/m for 5 days) then on 7th day a single I/M injection of 500 I.U. PMSG (Folligon).
- Check the estrus in the animal on 8th to 9th day.

OR

Rx

- GnRH analogue (Buseraline acetate, Receptal 5 ml) 20 μg I/M
- May be repeated after 10 days.
- Check the animal for estrus within few days.

OR

Rx

- GnRH analogue 20 μg I/M
- After 7 days, Lutalyse 25 mg I/M

- Observe the estrus in the animal and at the time of AI/NS on day 9th again inject GnRH analogue 20 μg I/M.

OR

Rx

- GnRH analogue 20 μg I/M
- Palpate the ovary for the presence of CL after 7 to 10 days, if there is CL then inject Lutalyse 25 mg I/M, If CL is not found then repeat GnRH analogue 20 μg I/M.
- Then observe the animal for estrus within few days.

OR

Rx

Insert Norgestomet Ear Implant (CRESTAR, Intervet), containing 3 mg norgestomet, in the outer surface of the ear for 9 days, also administer 2ml injection,i/m., containing 3mg norgestomet and 5mg estradiol valerate at the time of implant application. Then remove the implant. The animal will turn into estrus within 48 to 72 hrs after removal of implant.

OR

The animal may be fitted with CIDR (Controlled intravaginal drug release) device containing 1.38g progesterone (Ezibred, Livestock improvement, Hamilton, NewZealand) for 7- 8 days. Then remove the device. The animal will turn into estrus within 48 to 72 hrs after removal of device.

□□□

Case-3

A REPEAT BREEDER (CYCLIC NON-BREEDER) COW / BUFFALO

The animal is apparently normal but not conceiving inspite of 3 or more services (AI or NS) given and having no palpable abnormalities in the genitalia and regularly coming into estrus at 20-21 days interval. Repeat breeding is one of the most important problems the veterinarians face in the field. Farmers also get vexed to bring the animal repeatedly without knowing the future of the animal.

Causes

(a) Failure of fertilization

Ovulatory defects

Ovulation in the cow is atypical since it occurs 10-12 hr after the end of estrus and 24 after the onset of LH surge. The ovulatory defects may be due to endocrine deficiency or imbalance and mechanical factors.

i. Delayed ovulation

Certain cows have prolonged estrus and there may be lack of LH that is why the ovulation is delayed. It may be diagnosed by sequential rectal palpation of the ovaries e.g; at interval of 12 or 24 hr.

Treatment (Rx)

- GnRH analogue 20 μg I/M (Receptal 5 ml)

OR

- hCG 1500 I.U. (Chorulon) i/m or i/v.
- Repeat AI at 12-24 hr interval two times.

(Note: If the estrus duration in repeater cow is prolonged then shift the AI on 2nd or 3 rd day after the onset of estrus. In such cases AI is not advisable on Ist day)

ii. Anovulation

- May occur when the cow goes into anestrus or during the first cycle after parturition.
- Diagnosis of anovulation can be made retrospectively by noting on rectal palpation that a follicle persists longer than one would have suspected.
- Anovulatory follicle under goes luteinization and regresses like a normal CL after 17-18 days.

Treatment (Rx)

Same as described for delayed ovulations.

iii. Defects of the ovum

- Defective ovum
- Ageing of ovum – ova are viable for only few hours

% of ova fertilized	AI hrs. after ovulation
75	2-8
60	9-12
25	14-16
0	>24

iv. Inability of the sperm to fertilize a viable ovum

- High sperm abnormalities
- Low individual motility
- Low sperm concentration
- Inflammatory conditions of genital tract
- Very early AI or ageing of sperms

v. Inability of gametes to reach at site of fertilization

- Anatomical defects of genital tract with congenital and acquired.
- Segmental aplasia
- Tubal block
- Various affections of oviduct leading to obstruction.

(b) Early embryonic death

- Embryo loss accounts for the major portion of the reproductive wastage.
- The embryo death occurs gradually between days 8 and 18 after breeding.

- The embryo death most of the time occurs before the critical stage of pregnancy recognition i.e; the cow will return to estrus at the normal 20-25 days interval.

Causes

i. Unfavourable uterine environment

ii. Hormonal imbalance

iii. Infections (sub clinical endometritis)

iv. Negative energy balance

v. Environmental stress

Treatment (Rx)

i. Administration of LH (hCG) injection 1500 I.U. I/M at 3 to 4 days after AI.

(Note: The administration of hCG or GnRH during luteal phase converts small luteal cells into large luteal cells and thus enhances progesterone secretion from endogenous Corpus luteum and thus maintains the pregnancy).

ii. Sometimes the administration of 500 mg progesterone on 4th day of AI tends to increase the pregnancy rate.

iii. Intrauterine infusion of antibiotics like Lixen or Cflox TZ etc may preferably be tried, two to three times at the onset of estrus, or 8 hrs after AI and 24 hr later.

iv. 10 seconds stimulation of clitoris at A.I.

v. Ensure the animal into positive nutritive balance.

vi. Check the semen quality - use only high quality semen.

vii. Intrauterine infusion of 5 ml of Lugol's solutions diluted with 20 ml sterile distilled water and AI at next estrus.

viii. Flushing of the uterus with normal saline - under a moderate pressure (to remove cellular debris and also mild block in the uterine tubes).

ix. Supplementation of Vit E along with selenium and mineral mixture also helpful.

x. Now a days certain modern approaches (Alternative to antibiotic therapy) are also advised for good success rate:

   (a) I/U infusion of 40 to 50 ml of autologus blood plasma two times at 24 hr interval. (It enhances uterine defense mechanism as plasma contains immunoglobulins which acts as an opsonin and thus enhances phagocytosis and clears the infection from the uterus).

   (b) I/U infusion of 200 μg of E.coli LPS (Sigma Co.) dissolved into 20 ml distilled water & infused two times at 24 intervals. (It acts as chemoattractant, which results into more number of polymorphs infiltrate at the site of infection and thus provides cellular mediated immunity into the uterus).

Case-4

POST PARTUM CERVICO-VAGINAL PROLAPSE IN A COW / BUFFALO

The cervico - vaginal prolapse is the common problem in cows & buffaloes. The condition worsens with the time, therefore, early intervention is essential to replace the organs in position and to prevent it from further injury or damage.

Clinical Observations

The prolapsed mass may be dry, congested, inflammed, edematous and may be lacerated.

Treatment

(i) Reduction

- First attempt should be made to reduce the volume of prolapsed mass.
- Restrain the animal in standing position.
- Give epidural anesthesia (inject 5 to 10 ml of 2% Lignocaine /Xylocaine into the epidural space between last sacral & Ist coccygeal vertebrae).
- The urine may be drained by lifting the prolapsed mass above the inchial arch.

OR

- Evacuate the urinary bladder by passing the urinary catheter.
- The mass should be cleaned with 1:1000 potassium permanganate solution.
- Massage with warm saline water or sugar solution may be applied - to reduce edema of prolapsed mass.

(ii) Reposition

- Before attempting repulsion ensure no rupture of the tissue, if any laceration is seen then the lacerated area should be closed with continuous lambert sutures with horizontal mattress using chromic catgut (No.3).
- Raise the prolapsed mass to the level of ischial arch.
- Then the reduced mass should be repelled back into its normal position/original location by applying outside force with palm on the prolapsed mass.
- Once half portion will go inside then the rest half portion will go easily in a short time.

(iii) Retention

To prevent recurrence, rope truss may be applied.

Rope Truss Method

Pleace the rope truss over vulvar lips at appropriate location and hold it in position using rope tied around neck and shoulder. Ensure passage of urine.

Vulvar Suturing

(a) Lacing of vulva (using umbilical tape/nylon ribbon)

i. Suture vulva ensuring that the sutures are passing at least 2-3 inches lateral to the vulvar lips in the hair line.

ii. Use knots that can be easily untied or released when desired.

iii. Do antiseptic dressing, daily.

(b) Buhner's method (Burried or hidden purse string type of sutures)

i. The vulvar sutures are helpful particularly when the animal is straining too much.

ii. Inject 7-8 ml of 2% xylocaine epidurally

iii. Disinfect vulva and perineal region.

iv. Make 1 cm holizontal skin incision mid way between anus and dorsal commissure and 1.5 cm horizontal incision cranial to the normally projected ventral commissure.

v. Pass Buhner's needle through lower incision to dorsal incision and pass antibiotic soaked suture tape.

vi. Pass the antibiotics soaked suture tape on the upposite side also.

vii. Tighten the sutures in a way that permits entry of 2 to 3 fingers only.

Drugs

i. Give broad spectrum antibiotics like ampicillin or cloxacillin 2 gm i/m bid for 5 days

ii. Inj.Chlorphenaramine maleate 0.4 to 0.5 mg/kg body wt I/M once daily for 3-5 days

iii. Calcium preparations 200 to 450 ml subcut or i/v

iv. Inj Melonex 0.5 mg/kg body wt, I/M once daily for 3 days.

v. Straining of the animal gradually reduced and ceased after 3to4 days.

Precautions

i. Keep constant and close observation to the animal.

ii. Give laxative diet to the animal.

❑❑❑

Case-5

A COW / BUFFALO WITH RETAINED FETAL MEMBRANES (RFM)

- The fetal membranes, if retained in uterus beyond 12 hr after parturition, may cause uterine infection, infertility and sometimes steritity.
- Proper treatment and attention should be paid to avoid such undesired sequele of RFM.
- The incidence of RFM is quite variable, however, except in circumstances such as brucella infected herds, dystocias or nutritional deficiencies, the range is reported to be in between 7 to 12%.
- Temporary reduction of milk yield and impairment of appetite occurs in more than 70% of affected cows.

Consequences

i. An increase in calving to service interval.

ii. Increase in number of services per conception.

iii. Prolonged inter calving interval.

iv. Higher culling rate is observed due to metritis, and sometimes adhesions following RFM.

v. The cows which have suffered RFM are at significantly higher risk for developing mastitis, ketosis and others.

Treatment

(i) Manual Removal

It involved peeling of the cotyledons from carnucle with one hand and gentle traction of hanging mass using other hand. It should be attempted only after 72 or 96 hr post partum. Manual removal may result into severe damage to endometrium and inhibit the uterine defense mechanism.

(ii) Antibacterials

i. Give antibiotics like ampicillin 2 gm im or cloxacillin bid for 3-5 days.

ii. Inj. Chlorphenaramine maleate 0.4 to 0.5 mg/kg body wt I/M once daily for 3-5 days.

iii. Calcium preparations 200 to 450 ml subcut or i/v

iv. Inj Melonex 0.5 mg/kg body wt, I/M once daily for 3 days.

(ii) Administration of Ecbolic drugs

- Such as oxytocin,
- Estrogen,
- Ergot derivatives,
- Calcium preparations &

- Intrauterine insertion of antibacterials and antibiotics to control uterine infections.
- Injection of PGF_2alpha also expelled fetal membranes sooner and tender to have better reproductive performance in dairy cows.

Prevention of RFM

i. Provision of exercise alongwith administration of antioxidants like Selenium supplementation alone or with vitamin E and beta-carotene during 4 weeks before parturition i.e. during dry period.

ii. Use of oxytocin (30-50 IU) immediately after calving.

iii. PGF_2 alpha administration just following calving.

❐❐❐

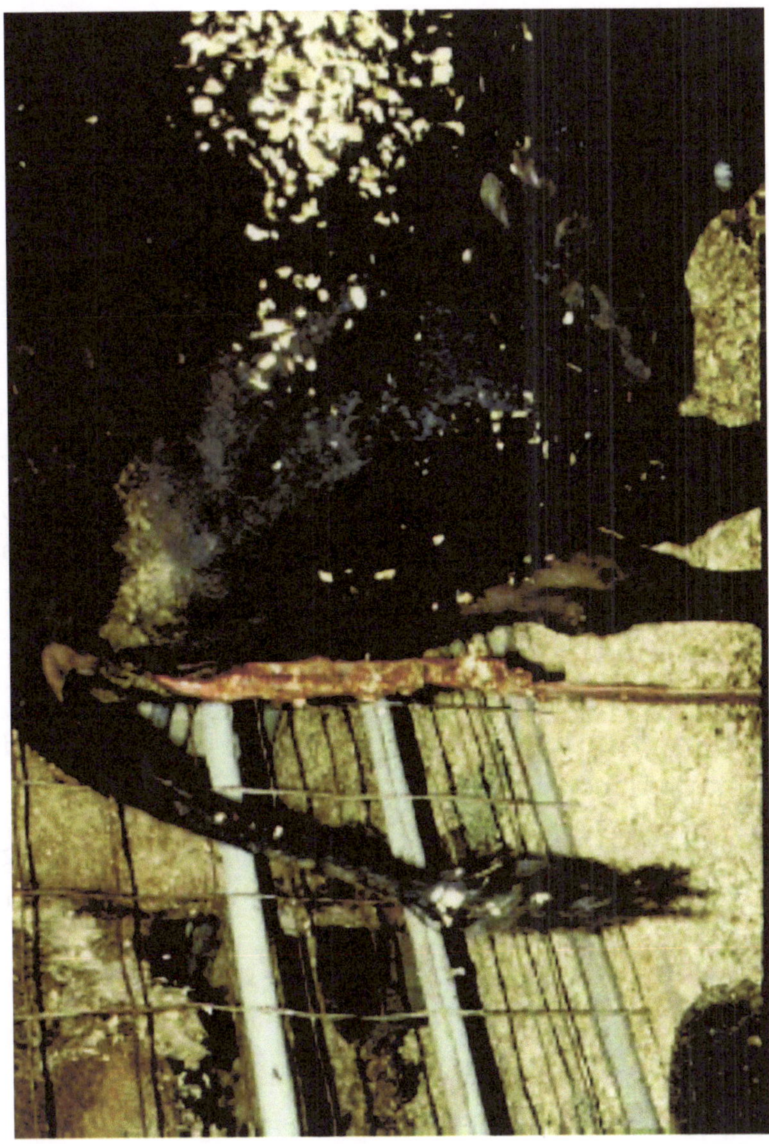

Plate - 3 : Retained Placenta in a Cow

Case-6

ENDOMETRITIS IN A COW / BUFFALO

- Endometritis is a common cause of infertility in dairy animals and is associated with uterine infection following abnormal parturitions eg; abortion, RFM, premature/still births, dystocia etc.
- The most common organisms responsible for uterine infection are C. pyogens, E. coli, Pseudomonas aeroginosa, streptococci and staphylococci.
- The infections in cows resulted in lochia assuming white, yellow white or grey mucopurulent character.

Treatment

An ideal therapy of uterine infection should

a. Eliminate bacteria from uterus

b. Not inhibit the normal uterine defense mechanism (UDM)

c. Not cause further adulteration of milk and meat for human consumption.

Rx

(i) Antibiotic therapy

(Any broad spectrum like Oxytetracycline, Cflox TZ or Lixen etc.)

- The success of IU treatment depends on absorption of the drug in the uterus. When the absorption of drug is low, therapeutic levels in the deeper layers of the uterus and other parts of the genital tract are not likely to be achieved. Therefore in this situation, the administration of drug should be done at frequent intervals.
- Furthermore, inrritating IU antibacterials should not be used in post partum dairy cows as might cause a necrotizing endometritis.
- Hence, systemic administration of antibiotic is fruitful in immediate postpartum cases.

Rx

(ii) PGF_2 α therapy

- PGF_2 α and its analogues have been widely used in endometritis & pyometra.
- The rationale of using PGF_2 α for uterine infections is

i. It induces luteolysis, decreases progesterone inhibition of UDM,

ii. Estrogen production, which follows luteolysis, stimulates the UDM,

iii. It may stimulate myometrial contractions that aid in the expulsion of uterine lochia, pus or other contents and

iv. It may have a stimulatory effect on phagocytosis by uterine levcocytes.

Rx

(iii) Immunomodulatory therapies

(a) I/U infusion of 40 to 50 ml of autologus blood plasma two times at 24 hr intervals. (It enhances uterine defense mechanism as plasma contains immunoglobulins which acts as an opsonin and thus enhances phagocytosis and clears the infection from the uterus).

OR

(b) I/U infusion of 200 μg of *E.coli* LPS (Sigma Co.) dissolved into 20 ml distilled water & infused two times at 24hr intervals. (It acts as chemoattractant, which results into more number of polymorphs infiltrate at the site of infection and thus provides cellular mediated immunity into the uterus).

OR

(c) I/U infusion of 40 to 50 ml of Neem oil two times at 24hr intervals (1ml of neem oil contains 1.1 mg of nimbidin which is equal to 500 IU of Penicillin and 5 mg of Streptomycin).It recovers the animals from endometritis and enhances conception rate.

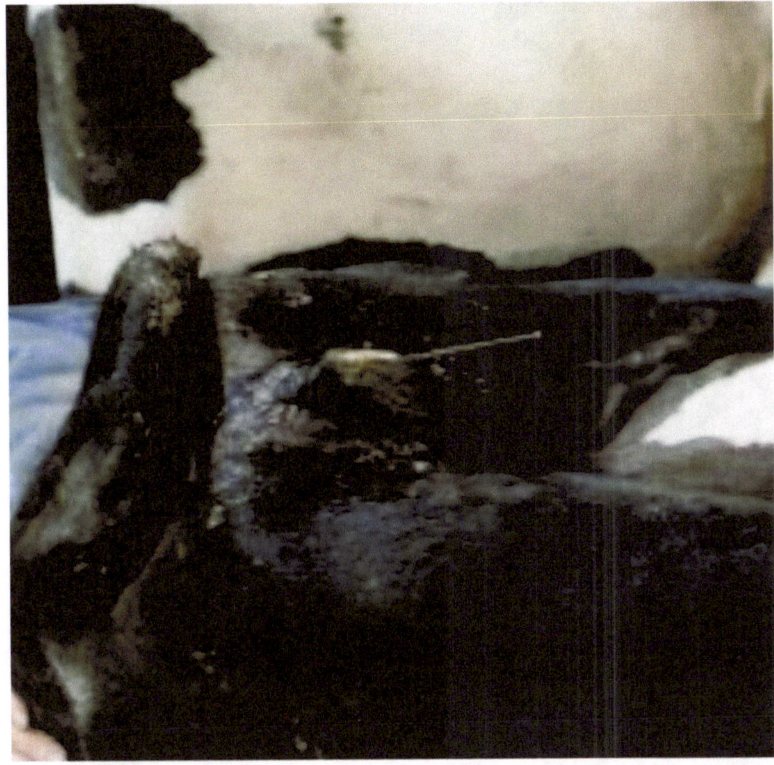

Plate - 4 : Endometritis in a Cow

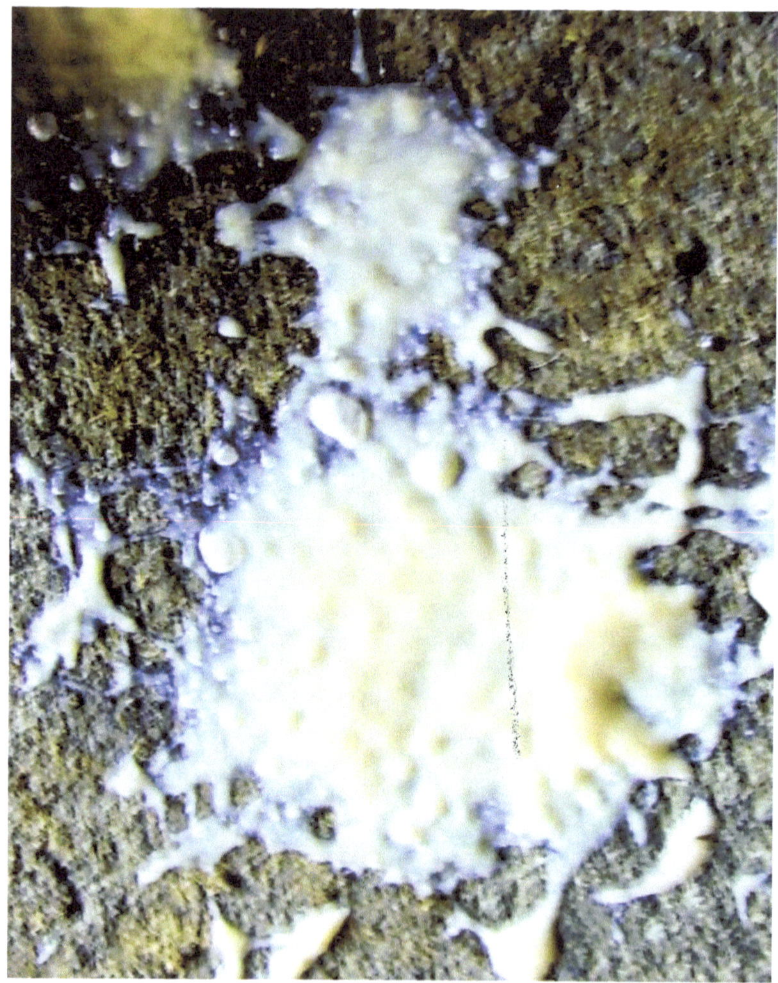

Plate - 5 : Discharge from a Metritic Cow

Case-7

SUB ESTRUS IN A BUFFALO

Silent heat or subestrus is used to indicate that ovulation has taken place but no external sign of estrus or often mild. The occurrence is common in milch buffaloes.

Causes

- Lack of sufficient secretion of estradiol hormone by the mature and secondary follicles of the ovary or due to need for higher threshold of estrogen for the Central nervous system to show the heat symptoms.

Diagnosis

- Based on clinical symptoms and other estrus signs like frequent micturition, temperament of animal etc.
- By rectal palpation, the presence of periodical normal CL in either of the ovary, this indicates occurrence of estrus & ovulation.

Treatment

i. To improve the estrus detection methods - Increase the frequency and duration of observation of the animals for estrus signs especially in early morning & late evening hrs.

ii. Careful & frequent examination of genital tract.

iii. Accurate maintenance of record.

iv. Supplementation of minerals & Vitamins or IVRI mineral mixture formulation

v. Fixed time of natural service or AI by using single injection of PGF_2 alpha or double injections at 11 days interval.

OR

Insert Norgestomet Ear Implant (CRESTAR, Intervet), containing 3 mg norgestomet, in the outer surface of the ear for 9 days, also administer 2ml injection,i/m., containing 3mg norgestomet and 5mg estradiol valerate at the time of implant application. Then remove the implant. The animal will turn into estrus with good behavioural signs within 48 to 72 hrs after removal of implant.

OR

The animal may be fitted with CIDR (Controlled intravaginal drug release) device containing 1.38g progesterone (Ezibred, Livestock improvement, Hamilton, NewZealand) for 7- 8 days. Then remove the device. The animal will turn into estrus with good visible signs within 48 to 72 hrs after removal of device.

❑❑❑

Case-8

CYSTIC OVARIAN DEGENERATION IN A CROSSBRED COW

Cystic ovarian degeneration (COD) is defined as persistence of an anovulatory follicular structure larger than 2.5 cm for more than 10 days, accompanied by cyclic irregularity in the absence of CL.

- Cystic ovaries are principally a disease of dairy cows due to improperly timed or inadequate Luteinizing hormone (LH) surge from pituitary.

Etiology

Season,

Hereditary,

Parity,

High Yield,

High Protein diet,

Administration of Steroids hormones,

Miscellaneous and unknown causes.

Symptoms

- Symptoms of follicular cysts are usually nymphomania.
- The nymphomanic cows ride on other cows but often refuse to stand to be ridden.
- Sterility hump i.e; tipping of pelvis due to relaxation of sacro - sciatic ligament.
- Adrenal virilism (steer like appearance).
- The genital organs are slightly edematous and atonic and mucus may be whitish grey in colour.

Diagnosis

- Based on clinical symptoms and history of short cycles with long duration of heat.
- Rectal examination of genitalia.One can find large size Table tennis ball like ovary and soft blister like fluid filled follicles therein.

Treatment

Main aim of treating the cyst is either to make it ovulate or to luteinize it.

Rx

i. Follicular cyst is treated with GnRH 20 μg (5 ml) I/M

   Or

   hCG 3000 I.U. to 5000 I.U. I/M.

ii. Luteal cyst is treated with $PGF_2\alpha$

iii. Many combinations are also used without differentiating whether the cyst is follicular or luteal eg; either hCG or GnRH injected and $PGF_2\alpha$ administered seven days later. The animal will return into estrus within 60 to 72 hrs of PG injection. It is advisable that breed the animal at subsequent estrus.

(*Note:* GnRH or LH causes luteinization of cyst where as administration of PGF_2 α 10 days later causes lysis of the luteinized cyst).

iv. Mineral supplementation along with vit E and Selenium is also found useful.

v. Corticosteroid therapy.

vi. Sometimes sexual rest for one or two cycles is also found beneficial in recovery of the animal, however, attention should be paid in chronic cases.

□□□

Case-9

CERVICITIS IN A COW/BUFFALO

- Inflammation of the cervix may occur due to chronic irritation.
- Chronic and severe irritation of cervix by caustic chemicals or pathogenic bacteria may sometimes lead to fibrosis and stenosis of cervix.
- Cervical stenosis may follow severe infection or trauma.

Causes

- Either due to faulty inseminating procedures
- Vaginal infections usually produce cervicitis, especially to the external os of the cervix.
- Associated with pneumovagina
- Sequele of some infectious reproductive diseases
- Unhygienic surroundings
- Unknown causes

Diagnosis

By Vaginal speculum examination

By Rectal examination

Treatment

i. Should be directed for removal of the cause of irritation, where cervicitis associated with endometritis/metritis usually responds to the treatments indicated for metritis.

ii. Douching of cervix and vagina with mild warm antiseptic solutions along with local antibiotics may be helpful in hastening recovery.

iii. Administration of iodine preparations.

iv. Sexual rest for two or more estrus period is advisable in cases of severe cervicitis.

❑❑❑

Case-10

KINKED CERVIX IN A COW

- It is the cervical abnormality; commonly seen in cattle & buffaloes under field conditions.
- In this case the cervical canal may be tortuous bent or even stenosed.
- It is very difficult to pass AI catheter without damage to the cervix.
- The condition may be due to subsequent fibrosis in previous parturition.
- It is felt like a firm cylindrical structure located at right angle to its usual position in heifers whereas, in cows cervix is hard, enlarged, indurated and may be fibrosed. However, the estrous cycle in these animals is regular with mucus discharge.

Treatment

- Since genetic nature of defect, the infertile heifers with kinked cervix should be culled from breeding programme.
- 10 IU of oxytocin µm can be injected in heifers and cows at about 15 minutes before insemination, some success may occur.

❒❒❒

Case-11

PYOMETRA IN A COW / BUFFALO

Accumulation of pus in uterus is called as pyometra. It may be of two types:

i. Post service or pre-partum pyometra &

ii. Post-partum pyometra

- Post-service pyometra is mainly due to *Trichomonas fetus* infection.
- The pyometra is associated with persistent CL in the ovary and failure of estrus due to suppression of endometrial luteolytic factor.
- True pyometra seldom recovers spontaneously.

Diagnosis

i. By history of a longer period of anestrus

ii. By rectal examination the uterine wall is usually thickened, flaccid and atonic.

Treatment

It should be aimed (i) to case lysis of the CL so that animal comes into estrus when UDM is more functional and active (ii) to evacuate the pus and (iii) to overcome the uterine infection.

Rx

- PGF_2 α is the best drug to treat pyometra.

  (Note: It causes luteolysis, dilatation of cervix and contraction of uterus hence the pus inside the uterus can be evacuated).

- The treatment may be repeated after 10 days, if required.
- The cervix will be relaxed slowly within 5-6 days.
- Oxytocin 40-60 units a day later may be given for hastening expulsion of pus.

  Followed by parental antibiotics for 3 days.

❑❑❑

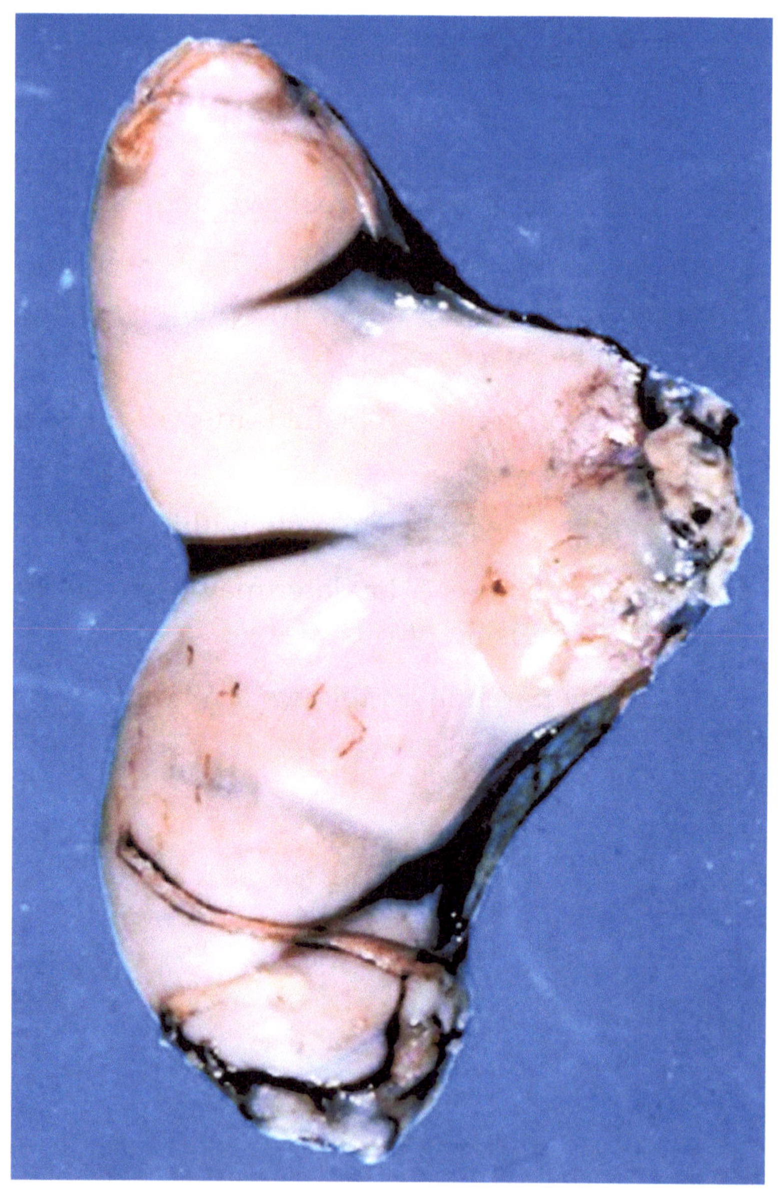

Plate - 6 : Buffalo Uterus filled with pus

Case-12

ABORTION IN A COW / BUFFALO

Each case of abortion should be examined for infectious causes like Brucellosis, Vibriosis, Trichomoniasis etc.

(A) Brucellosis

- Caused by *Brucella abortus*
- Characterized by abortion in last trimester of pregnancy and a subsequent period of infertility.

Etiology

- Contagious disease, spreads mainly through the ingestion of contaminated genital discharge, penetration through mucus membrane and intrauterine insemination with infected semen.
- Once established in pregnant animal it causes severe pathological changes in placenta results in abortion.
- After abortion the organism disappears for 1-5 months from uterus but persists in mammary gland and lymph nodes.

Diagnosis

- History of abortion in later part of pregnancy, ROP etc.
- Serum agglutination test
- Materials from suspected cases like placenta, genital discharge, fetal stomach contents or milk should be sent to laboratory for confirmatory diagnosis.

Treatment

- Costly & rarely successful.
- Once the organisms are located in the uterus their multiplication can not be prevented by medical treatment.
- Symptomatic treatment with tetracycline or streptomycin in high doses for long period can be carried out.

Prevention

- By calfhood vaccination of female calves at 6-9 months age with S-19 vaccine administration.
- Positive reactors in a herd should be culled and
- Semen from *Brucella* - free bulls should be used for AI.

The chart below provides an estimate of age for an aborted fetus:

Length of gestation	Description of fetus
Two months	Size of mouse
Three months	Size of rat
Four months	Size of small cat
Five months	Size of large cat
Six months	Size of small dog (hair around eyes, tail, muzzle)
Seven months	Fine hair on body and legs
Eight months	Hair coat complete, incisor teeth slightly erupted
Nine months	Incisor teeth erupted

(B) Vibriosis

- Caused by *Vibrio fetus veneralis.*
- Spread at the time of coitus or AI.
- Characterized by endometritis, early embryonic mortality, abortion at 4-7 months of gestation and infertility.

Diagnosis

- By clinical signs.
- Vaginal mucus agglutination test in a herd.
- Materials to be sent to laboratory for investigation are aborted fetal lung, stomach contents.

Treatment

- Not very reliable.
- The infected males should be culled.
- The disease can be controlled by AI with semen from bulls known to be free from Vibriosis under strict hygienic precautions.

(c) Trichomoniasis

- Caused by *Trichomonas fetus*.
- Characterized by early to mid stage abortion, pyometra and infertility.
- Moderate vulvo - vaginitis and cervicitis may be observed.
- Vaginal mucosa become rough & corrugated.

Diagnosis

- Following abortion, the organism disappears in the fetal membranes, stomach contents of fetus or exudate in the uterus within 48 hrs.
- By examining fresh samples for presence of organism.
- By clinical signs.

Treatment

- Affected animals are carrier for indefinite period.
- They may be segregated, treated with antibiotics & antiprotozoal drugs.
- Bred animals only by AI.
- Sexual rest is advised.

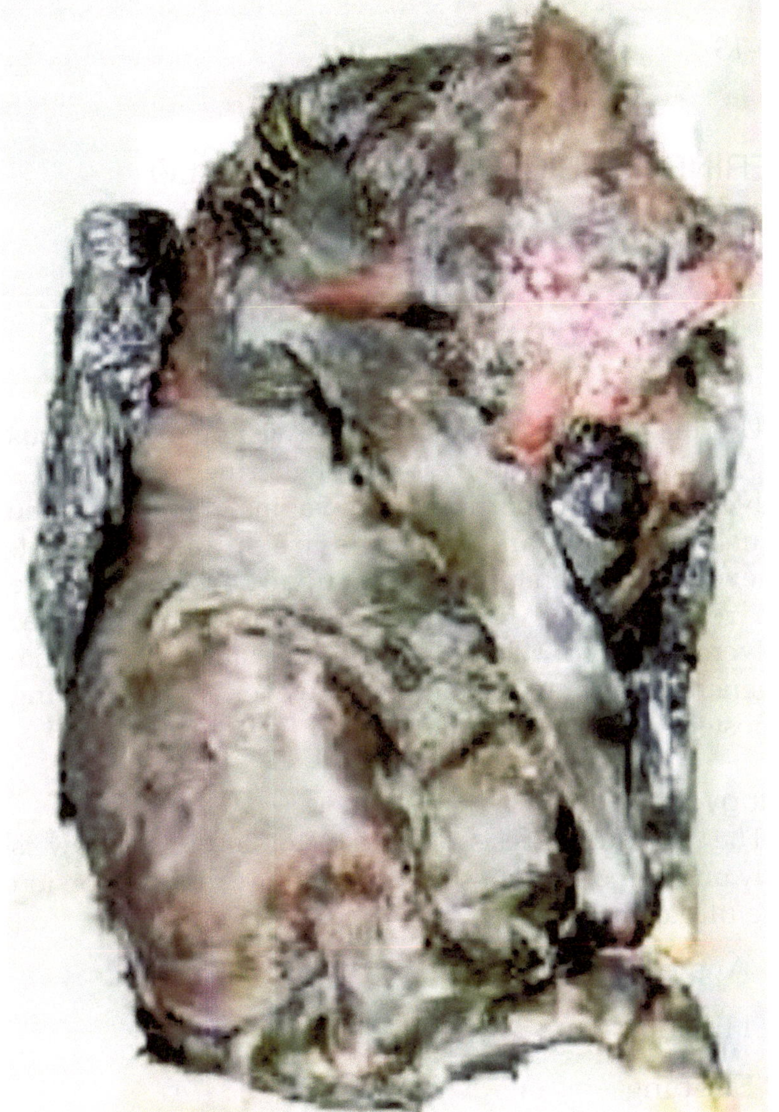

Plate - 7 : Aborted fetus at an later stage

Case-13

UTERINE TORSION IN A COW/BUFFALO

Uterine torsion is defined as the twisting of the uterus along its long axis. The majority of uterine torsion cases involve the cephalic portion of the vagina. Stenosis of the vagina is present, and its walls are spirally twisted. However, it has been reported that up to 34% of cases have been recognized to be precervical with no vaginal involvement noted. When the twist does affect the vagina, it is generally the anterior vagina. However, cases involving the posterior vagina do occur.

Etiology

The etiopathogenesis of uterine torsion in the cow is poorly understood. Proposed contributing causes for torsion of the uterus include:

- Anatomy of the cow
- Hilly terrain
- Slipping
- Butt in the flank from another cow
- Manner in which the cow rises

- Stabling a cow
- Energetic movements of the fetus during first stage labor
- Deep capacious abdomen
- Lack of tone to the uterus
- Lack of fetal fluids
- Reduced rumen volume prior to parturition
- Wallowing behaviour in buffaloes

Clinical Signs and Symptoms

The main clinical signs are as follows:

- Tachycardia (93%)
- Tachypnea (94%)
- Fever (23%)
- Straining (23%)
- Decreased rumen activity
- Constipation
- Restlessness
- Tail switching
- Treading
- Abdominal pain

Dignosis

i. By rectal examination: The broad ligaments can be felt to be crossed and the uterus twisted. The vulva can often be seen to have a slight twist of the dorsal portion.

ii. By vaginal examination: Vaginal palpation should also be performed with a suspected uterine torsion. The vaginal wall can be felt to be twisted or spiraled. This can be visualized with the aid of a speculum. Folds in the vaginal wall will indicate the direction of the torsion. For instance, in a counterclockwise torsion, folds of the dorsum vagina spiral downwards and forward to the left. It is suggested that a rectal palpation always be performed in suspected cases even if not torsion is felt vaginally. Occasionally the twisted portion of the uterus may lie near the body of the uterus and not extend into the vagina. However, as stated previously, the majority of cases in the bovine do involve the cephalic vagina.

Treatment

i. Rolling of dam towards the same side of torsion (By Shaffer's Method)

ii. Rotation of dam

iii. By laparohysterotomy: Anytime the torsion is irreducible or the cervix refuses to dilate, surgical correction is often a requirement. Surgical correction is also indicated when the cervix has undergone secondary constriction after prolonged dystocia with an emphysematous fetus.

The image on the left represents the normal position of the uterus with a left horn pregnancy. The image on the right represents torsion to the right.

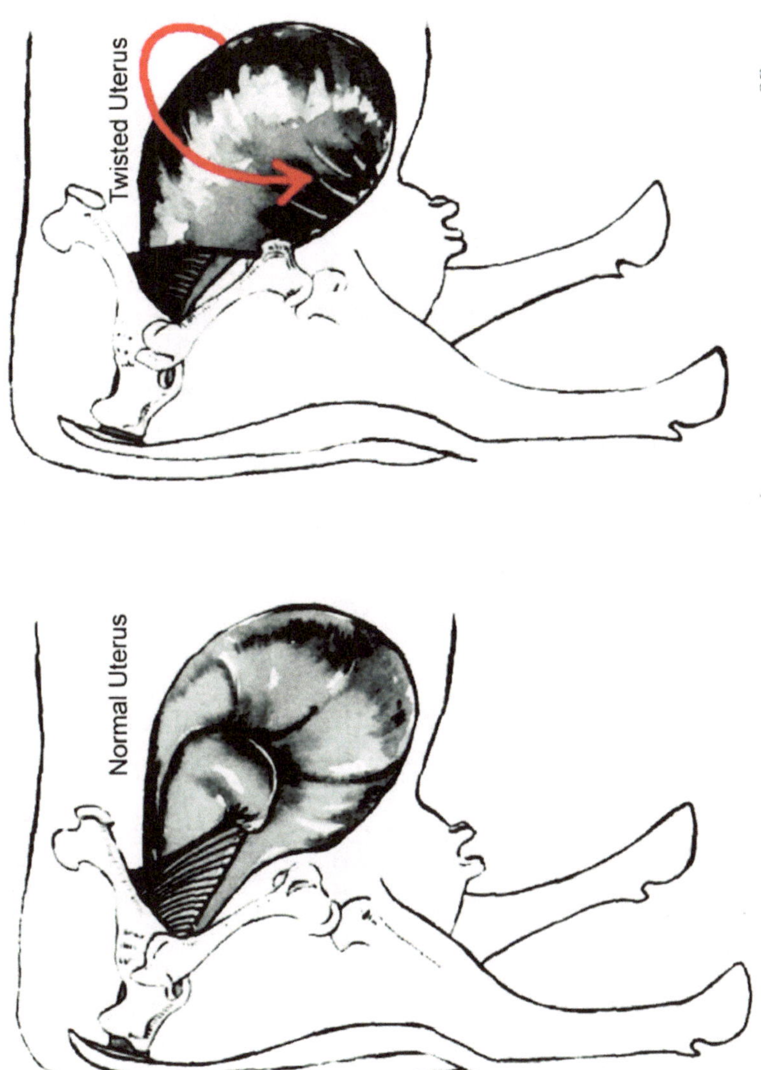

Fig. 1 : The representation of the occurrence of a uterine torsion in a cow

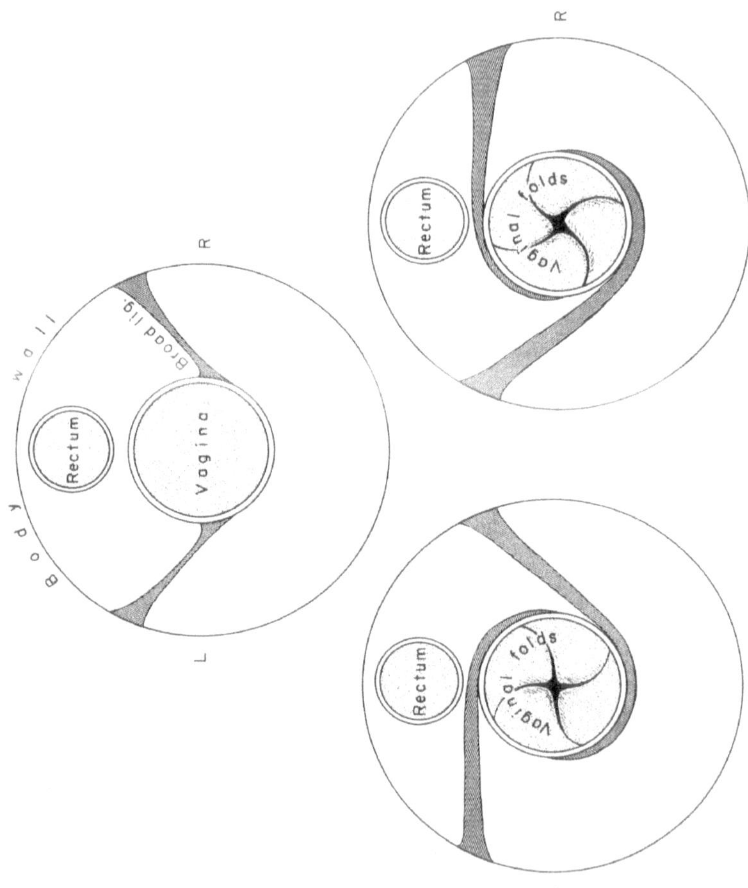

Fig. 2 : Represents a comparison of a normal and twisted bovine uterus

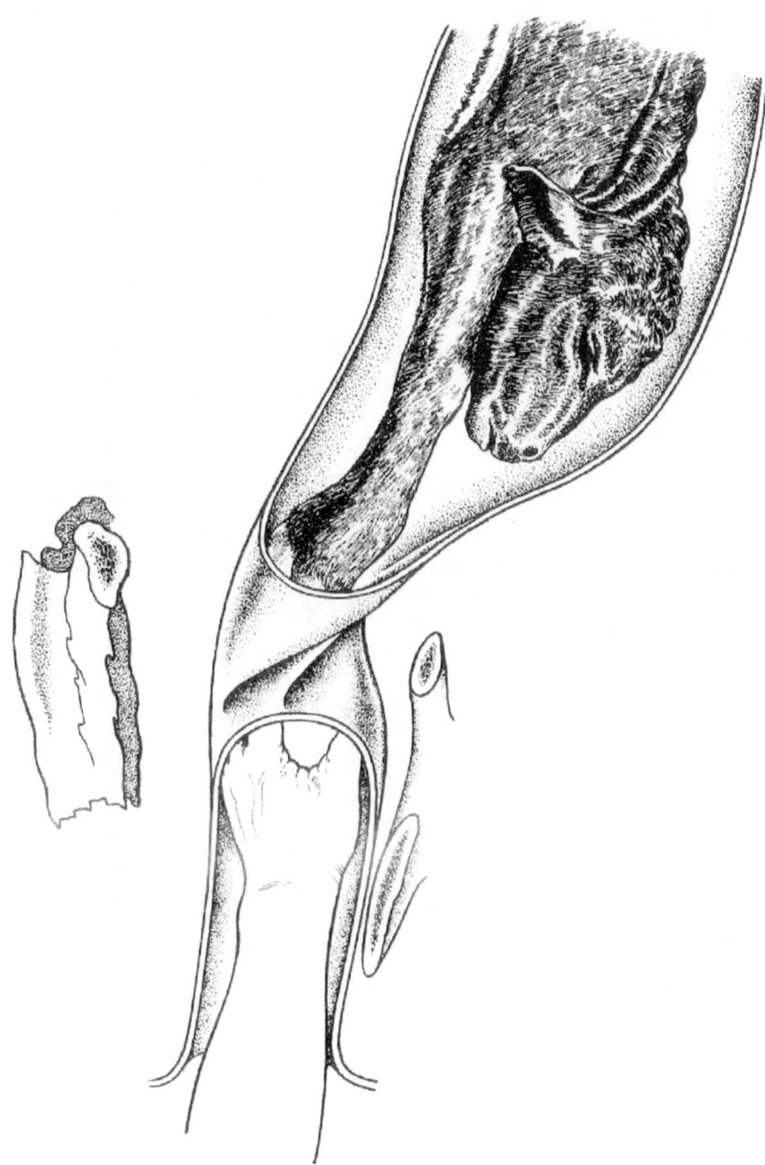

Fig. 3 : Vaginal examination of torsion

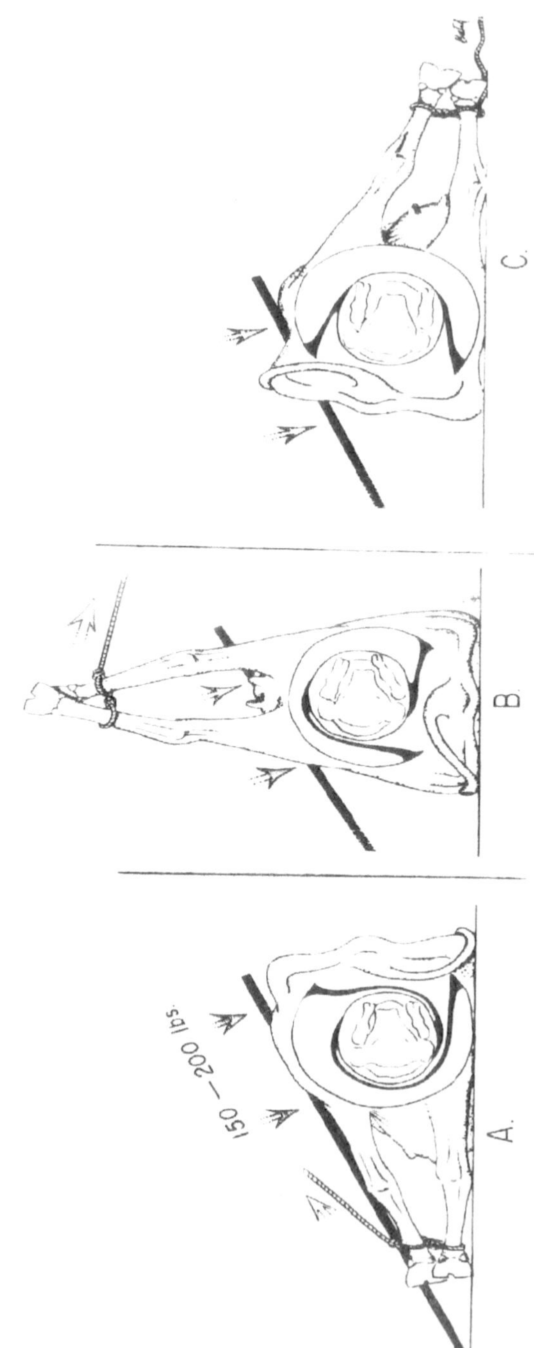

Fig. 4 : Shaffer's Method for Correction of uterine Torsion

Case-14

DETERMINE THE CORRECT TIMING OF A.I. IN COW / BUFFALO

- The estrus period is short in the cow i.e. 12-24 hours.
- Ovulation occurs 10-12 hours after the end of estrus.
- Best conception rates occur if insemination is done in the middle to the end of the standing estrus i.e. 12-18 hours before ovulation.
- A cow that is first seen in estrus in the afternoon is to be inseminated in the next morning.
- While a cow seen in estrus in early morning, is inseminated in the afternoon of the same day.

Note: The accurate estrus signs for right time insemination should be observed on the basis of following points.

I. The fern pattern of cervicovaginal mucous :
   - Aspirated mucous is smeared on clean and wax free dry slide and allowed to dry at room temperature.
   - Arborization is visualized/ matched with the stage of the estrus/suitability of time of AI under microscope or in IVRI crystoscope available in the

market (Lyka exports, Ranbaxy India Limited, Cattle Remedies India Ltd. etc.)

II. Combined with other signs of estrus, typical fern pattern (crystallization) can be used as an aid to determine the proper time of insemination in field conditions.

III. The symptoms like frequent micturition, reddening of vulva with increased activity of animals, can be guiding factor for deciding time of insemination particularly in buffaloes under field conditions, where the estrus detection by teaser bull is not practiced.

❐❐❐

Canines

CHAPTER 4

Common Reproductive Problems in Canines

Case-1

CONTRACEPTION DUE TO MISALLIANCE AND TERMINATION OF PREGNANCY IN BITCHES

- It is obvious that breeders maintain varieties of breeds but mismating do occur within their own premises and sometimes by unwarranted stray animal.
- Misalliance complicates too many other problems.
- Incidence of mismating is 15 to 20 percent in canine breeding.

History regarding the mismating or misalliance generally involves

i. Sudden at day '0' of the Estrous cycle.
ii. Delayed report at days 7th to 14th of the O.C.
iii. Confirmed report after 3 to 4 weeks after mating.

Diagnosis

- Based on history (only gives a outline)
- For confirmation the various tests to be employed in the canine reproduction

1. Cytohumoral or cornification index

- Vaginal cytology with a help of sterile ear swab to rule out the cytological changes after staining with either Leishmans or Giemsa stain.
- The presence of the increasing trend of non-nucleated cornifying cells and the superficial cells as compared to intermediate and the parabasal cells with more RBC's indicating the estrus than that of the metestrus, diestrus and anestrus where more of parabasal and intermediate cells with almost no cornified cells and RBC's and occasional leucocytes may be noticed.

2. Presence of Sperms

In the vaginal cavity either by taking a vaginal swab or by aspiration of the contents in one ml of saline to rule out the presence of cornified cells mixed along with the sperms, if the mating has occurred within 12 to 24 hrs.

3. Progesterone assay

After day 10 post estrus or post coital period to rule out the elevation of more than 2 ng/ml of progresterone which can be estimated by RIA or EIA.

4. Trans-abdominal Ultrasonography

After four weeks of gestation for the presence of distention in the uterus and ecogenic mass extending in both the uterine cornua.

Control Measures

Treatment with hormones and other related drugs:

(i) Estrogen therapy

This therapy should be combined with haematinics and antibiotics:

Dose of E_2: Single I/M injection of 0.1 mg/kg body weight. (Prygynon depot - 1ml amp available)

This is 100% effective within 4 to 7 days of mismating.

Mode of Action

- Increases the level of estrogen, which prolongs the estrus period and delays the ovulation, leading to the failure of fertilization.
- Interfere with transport of zygote by tightening the uterotubular function and prolong oviductal retention, thus preventing migration into the uterus.

- The effect of estrogen is directly an embryo toxic and causes a decline of estrogen: progesterone ratio.

(ii) Prostaglandin therapy

In case of delayed misalliance after a week or 10 days to any stage of gestation.

Dose: $PGF_2\alpha$ (Natural) 150 to 250 µg/kg body wt. sub cut daily for 3 days.

$PGF_2\alpha$ (Synthetic) 250 µg/kg body wt. sub cut twice a day for 3 to 4 days until the abortion complete.

Supportive therapy : Atropine @ 0.5 mg/ kg body wt I/M prior to $PGF_2\alpha$ treatment.

Mode of Action

It destroys the CL e.g; luteolysis & death of the fetus due to anoxia & expulsion of the conceptus as a result of increasing myometrial contractions acting as an ecbolic and abortifacient.

Adverse Reaction

Excess panting, salivation, emesis, respiratory distress, diarrhea, tachycardia etc. Therefore, if these symptoms occur then Avil or Phenargan or Indomethacin drugs are advised as an antidote to nullify the side effects of PG.

(iii) Dopamine agonist agents

Prolactin is the primary LH in dogs and is required for sustenance of the corpus luteum, which produces progesterone. When drugs that stimulate dopamine (Dopamine agonists) such as Bromocriptine or Cabergoline, are administered to the pregnant bitch during this prolactin increase, abortion occurs.

- A prolactin suppressing drug (Bromocriptine or Cabergoline)
- Ergot alkaloids

Dose: 5 μg/kg body wt orally twice daily for 5 days at 25 to 40 days of mating.

Side Effects

Anorexia, vomiting, depression, hence advise atropine type drug.

(iv) Glucocorticoids

Dose : Dexamethasone 0.5 mg / kg body wt I/M every 12 hr for 10 days beginning at day 35 or 40 of pregnancy or when given orally 2-3 times a day for 5 days followed by gradual reduction of dose over the following 3-5 days.However, this treatment is not recommended until further information is obtained.

Mode of Action

It initiates fetal death by increasing endogenous PGF levels resulting into luteolysis.

(v) Mifepristone: Ru 486

A Progesterone receptor antagonist induces abortion in 3 to 6 days.

Dose: 2.5 mg/kg Body wt BID from the day 30th of pregnancy.

Advise

- Give with hematinics & antibiotics.
- Use of IV fluids, if any side effects (vomition etc) appear.

❑❑❑

Case-2

TRANSMISSIBLE VENEREAL TUMOR IN A BITCH

- Naturally occurring tumor/growth.
- Affects external genitalia of either sex.
- Transmissible venereal tumor occurs via transplantation of neoplastic cells on to vaginal mucosa during coitus and on to nasal and oral mucosa by licking of affected genitalia of self or other dogs.

Diagnosis

(i) By History

Bleeding from external genitalia after mating.

(ii) By clinical signs

Sero-sanguinous discharge, licking of external genitalia and Protrusion of mass.

(iii) By vaginal examination

- With gloved, lubricated fingers, a pedunculated cauliflower like mass could be felt on caudo - dorsal aspect of posterior vagina.

- It may be a multilobular hemorrhagic mass approximately 5 cm in diameter.
- Impression smear reveals confirmatory diagnosis and TVT cells with prominent chromatin clumping, large nucleoli and large nucleus: cytoplasm ratio.

Treatment

Chemotherapeutic agents

i. Cyclophosphamide

ii. Vincristine sulphate

Dose

- 0.025 mg/kg Body wt i/v.
- Repeat after 2 weeks, if required.
- Tab. Emidoxyn 1 mg/kg Body wt (To avoid vomiting).
- Any Broad spectrum antibiotic orally Bid.
- If success not occurs then advise Radiation therapy.

❑❑❑

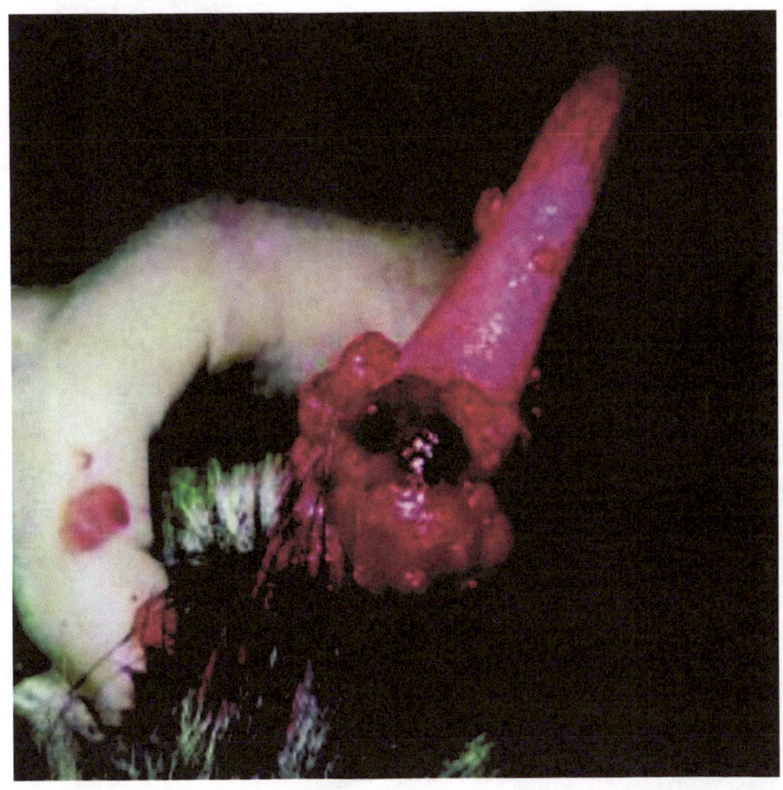

Plate - 8 : TVT in a male dog

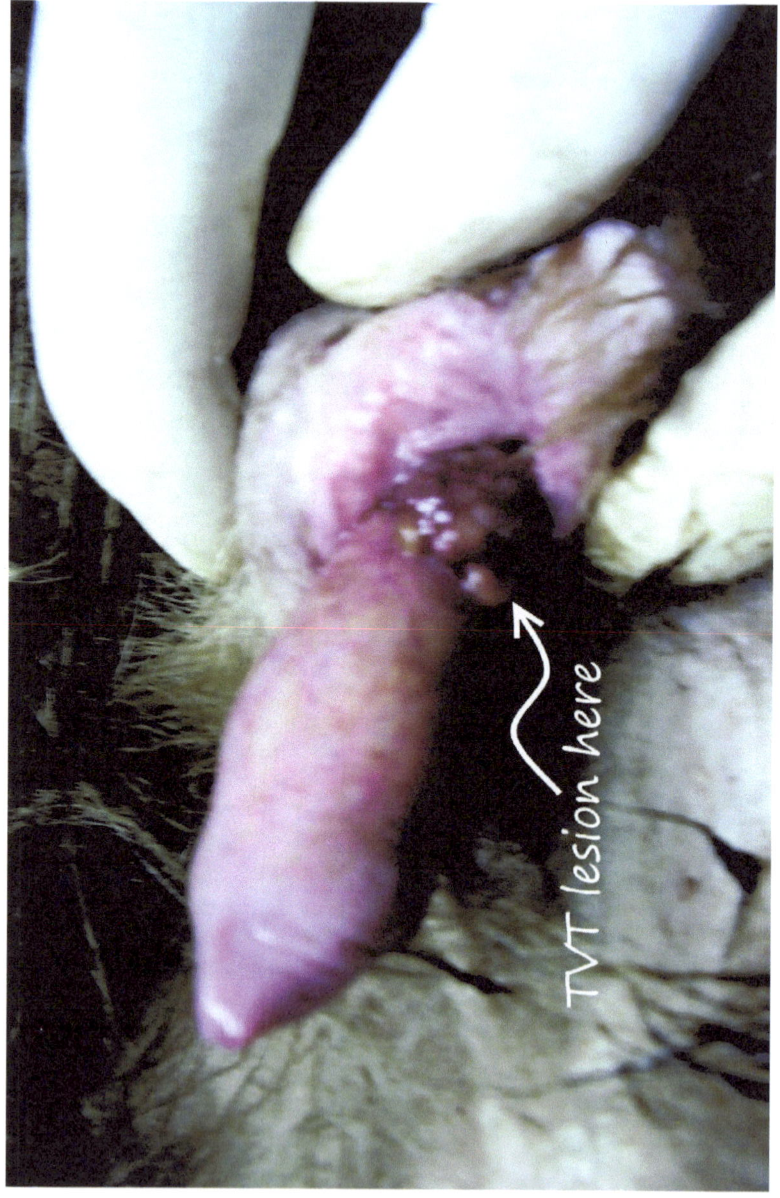

Plate - 9 : TVT in a male dog

Case-3

INDUCTION OF ESTRUS IN BITCHES

Nutritional deficiencies should be ruled out before deciding any hormonal treatments.

Treatments

1. *Antiprolactin drugs:* This is the most reliable and successful method Cabergoline (CABG)

   OR

   Bromocriptine during luteal please

Dose: 5 to 10 µg/ kg body wt bds for 5 to 7 days. Success occurs within 3 to 4 weeks.

2. PMSG + hCG

   PMSG 25 I.U. per kg body wt for 5days & on day 5th hCG (25 IU/ kg body wt)

3. GnRH

   Pulsatile administration of GnRH to anestrus bitches every 90 minutes for 6-8 days induce a fertile estrus. But this treatment is costlier.

4. Low doses of Estradiol

   5 mg daily orally diethyl stilboestrol for 7 to 10 days. If no response then increase the dose up to 10 mg for another 7 days.

❑❑❑

Case-4

DETECTION OF ESTRUS FOR OPTIMUM BREEDING TIME BY EXFOLIATIVE VAGINAL CYTOLOGY IN BITCHES

Examination of vaginal cytology is commonly used to monitor the O.C. in bitch and to determine the optimal time for mating or insemination.

Vaginal Cytology

- Collection of vaginal mucus and preparation of smear
- Air dry the smear
- Stain by Leishman's or Geimsa stain
- Observe the cells under oil immersion objective of microscope
- One can find different cells proportions during different stages of cycle as described below:

  In Proestrus : Large intermediate cells, superficial cells with dirty back ground and excessive RBCs.

  At Estrus : Superficial cornified cells are predominant, with clear back ground and inconsistent numbers of RBCs.

At Diestrus : Very few superficial, some intermediate and large amount of parabasal cells are found. WBCs are also seen in some cases.

At Anestrus : Large number of intermediate cells & parabasal cells. Neutrophils are predominant in this phase.

Remarks : For fertile breeding time in bitches: Higher percentage of superficial cells (90%), lower intermediate (7%) and parabasal cells (3%) at estrus.

This technique can be used efficiently in bitches and mating can be planned accordingly and may also be used in bitches with conception problem due to mating at improper time.

❑❑❑

Case-5

INDUCTION OF WHELPING IN BITCHES

- Parturition is a physiological process involved in expulsion of normal viable fetuses from the uterus through the maternal passage by natural forces alone at a stage when the young one is capable of independent existence.
- When parturition is delayed beyond the normal length it is called prolonged gestation.
- In longer gestation period a professional advice should be taken since with prolonged gestation fetal and maternal death can take place.

Diagnosis

- History of breeding,
- Ultrasonographic examination,
- X-ray examination,
- Presence of fully developed fetuses.

Treatment

- Depending on body wt (20 to 30 kg)
- Inj DNS 100 to 200 ml I/V
- Inj Calcium sandoz 20 ml to 40 ml I/m
- Inj Dexona 1 to 2 ml
- Wait for 8 to 12 hr.
- If delivery is not occur then use injections of Oxytocin (10 -20 I.U.) at intervals to aid in easy expulsion of pups.

❑❑❑

Case-6

MEDICAL MANAGEMENT OF CRYPTORCHIDISM IN PUPS

- Cryptorchidism in dogs refers to failure of one or both testes to descend into the scrotum by eight weeks of age.
- The incidence of cryptorchidism in dogs has been reported to range from 0.8 to 15 percent.

Treatment

For dogs of 12 to 16 weeks of age Inj 750 I.U. human Chorionic gonadotropin (hCG) 4 times during a two week period.

Remarks

i. There will be complete descent of the testes following treatment.

ii. Owners are advised not to breed these animals because of genetic implication.

❒❒❒

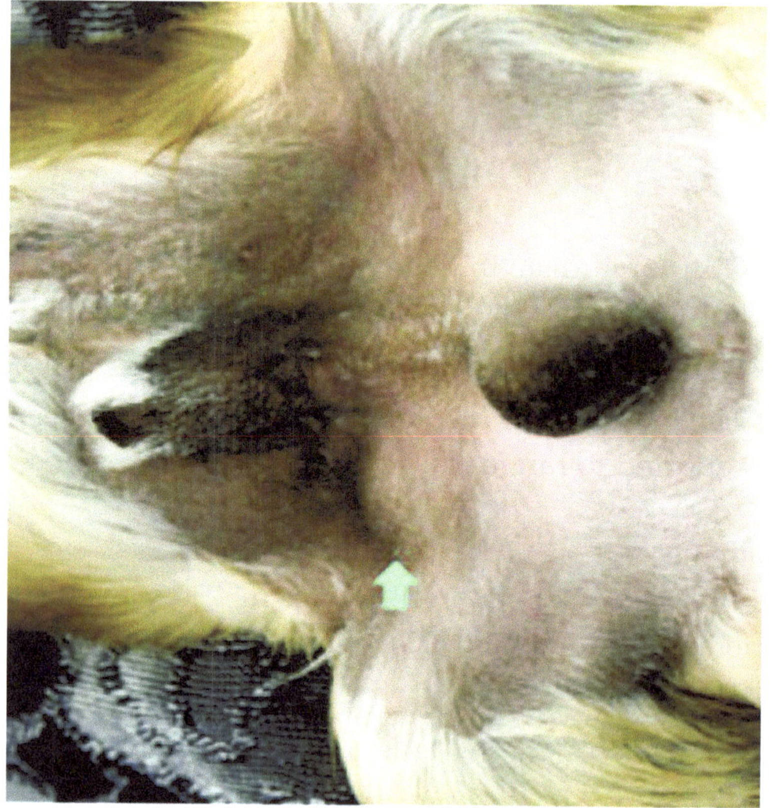

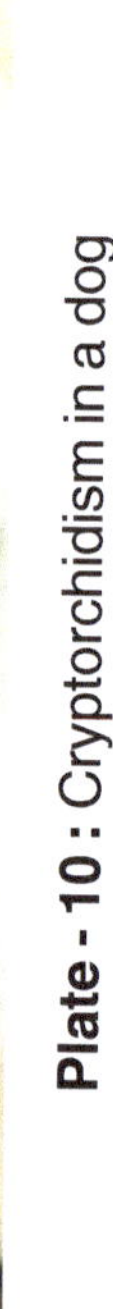

Plate - 10 : Cryptorchidism in a dog

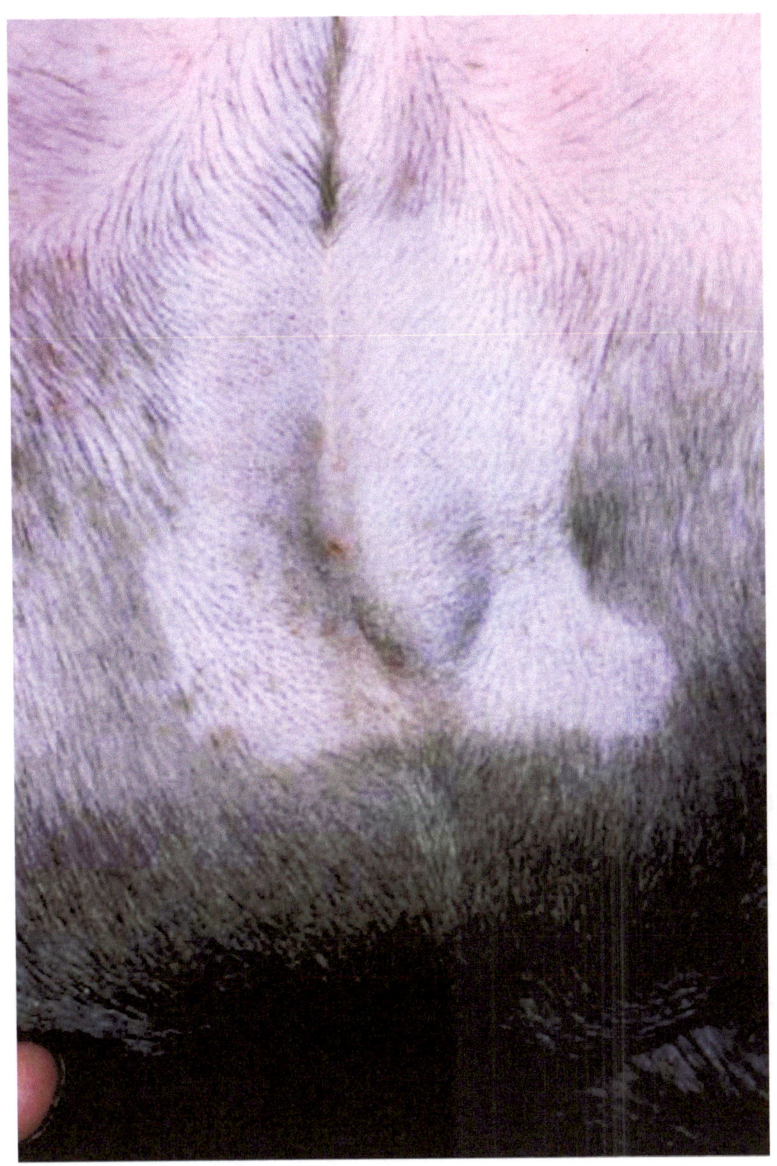

Plate - 11 : Inguinal cryptorchidism in a dog

Case-7

PYOMETRA IN A BITCH

- Pyometra is a disease of the luteal phase of the O.C. with most bitches showing clinical signs between 5 and 80 days after the end of estrus.
- It is relatively a common reproductive emergency in the nonpregnant middle aged & olds bitches.
- More commonly found in nulliparous bitches.

Causes

i. Infections

ii. Endocrine status

Diagnosis

Types : Closed cervix & open cervix pyometra.

i. *Based on clinical signs:* elevated temperature discharge coming out of the genital tract, anorexia, vomition, diarrhea, perineal soiling, and polydypsia.

ii. *Hematological parameters* : Decline in hemoglobin, neutrophlilia, elevated levels of BUN and creatinine.

iii. *By X-ray* : Reveals a homogenous ground glass appearance of ut. horns (In case of closed cervix pyometra).

iv. *By Ultrasonography:* In luteal phase by ultrasound examination of the uterus; (a) the presence of anechoic sacculations and (b) the detection of multiple, small, focal, fluid filled cystic regions within the endometrium – It leads to pyometra.

Treatment

i. Adequate fluid & electrolyte therapy.

ii. Antiprolactin drugs like Bromocriptine or Cabergoline @ 5 mg/kg body wt os daily for 7 days.

iii. Broad spectrum antibiotics like ciprofloxacin or cephalosporin I/M for 7 days.

iv. $PGF_2\alpha$ in tapering doses (150 to 250 μg/kg body wt) I/M for 7 days.

v. Supportive therapy.

vi. Combination of Mifipristone (Antiprogestine) 10 mg/kg body wt/day orally for three days and 10μg/kg body wt $PGF_2\alpha$ sub/cut twice a day for 5-7 days.

vii. Last therapy is to perform Ovariohysterectomy.

Note : There are some adverse effects of prostaglandin treatment, which may be noticed during 30 minutes immediately after the administration of PGF_2a, which included retching, vomiting, abdominal straining, diarrhea and panting.

❏❏❏

Case-8

CLINICAL MANAGEMENT OF PSEUDO-PREGNANCY IN BITCHES

Occasionally following the estrous cycle, a bitch that was either bred or not bred during estrus develops overt signs associated with pregnancy and lactation. If the bitch was bred, these signs may misguide the breeder to confirm a successful mating.

Symptoms

Complicating the situation further, around day 60 of the 'suspected' pregnancy, the bitch will often experience a decrease in body temperature and display enlargement of the mammary gland with secretion of milk, behavioral symptoms like nesting, restlessness, loss of appetite, vomiting and panting behaviour typical of a bitch about to whelp. However, no puppies will be delivered because the bitch is experiencing a condition known as pseudopregnancy.

Diagnosis

i. Thorough clinical examination - found normal

ii. Pregnancy diagnosis

- By physical Palpation
- Confirmation by ultrasound
- And if found to be nonpregnant then the condition may be diagnosed as pseudopregnancy.

Treatment

Bromocriptine or Cabergoline that blocks effects of prolactin may be used @ 5 µg/kg body wt of daily for 7 days.

Remarks

- There will be significant regression of mammary gland with cessation of milk and restoration of normal appetite after 7 days of treatment.
- There may be side effects like transient vomition etc, which can be treated symptomatically.

❑❑❑

Case-9

VAGINAL PROLAPSE IN A BITCH

- A vaginal mass protruding out from the vulva.
- Clinical examination revealed that the entire circumference of vagina may prolapsed to an extent of 3 to 4 inches or more out of the vulva, which may edematous, soft and pink in colour.
- Sometimes in delayed cases some necrotic area or severe inflammation can be noticed on the surface of prolapsed mass.

Treatment

(i) Reduction

- Before during reduction of prolapsed mass the vulva and perivulvar area thoroughly cleansed with an antiseptic solution and the protruded prolapsed mass should be cleaned with the help of normal saline solution.
- The urinary catheter should be passed in urinary bladder to evacuate it.

- The ice cubes should be applied over it and gently massaged to reduce swelling.
- Apply Lignocaine hydrochloride gelly.

(ii) Reposition

The prolapsed mass should be repositioned i.e. back in position. Take time in this operation. Once half portion goes inside then rest half will go easily.

(iii) Retention

- Apply two mattress sutures over vulval lips under local infiltration of 2% lignocaine hydrochloride.
- Parentally administer:
- Pheneramine maliate @5 mg / kg body wt
- Broad spectrum antibiotics like ampicilin @ 5-10 mg/kg body wt for 5 days.
- Progesterone @ 250 mg I/M on alternate days for 3 days.
- Calcium preparations like calcium sandoz 30 to 50 ml

OR

- Calcium borogluconate 30 to 50 ml i/v or sub/ cut.
- Sutures may be removed after a week of treatment.

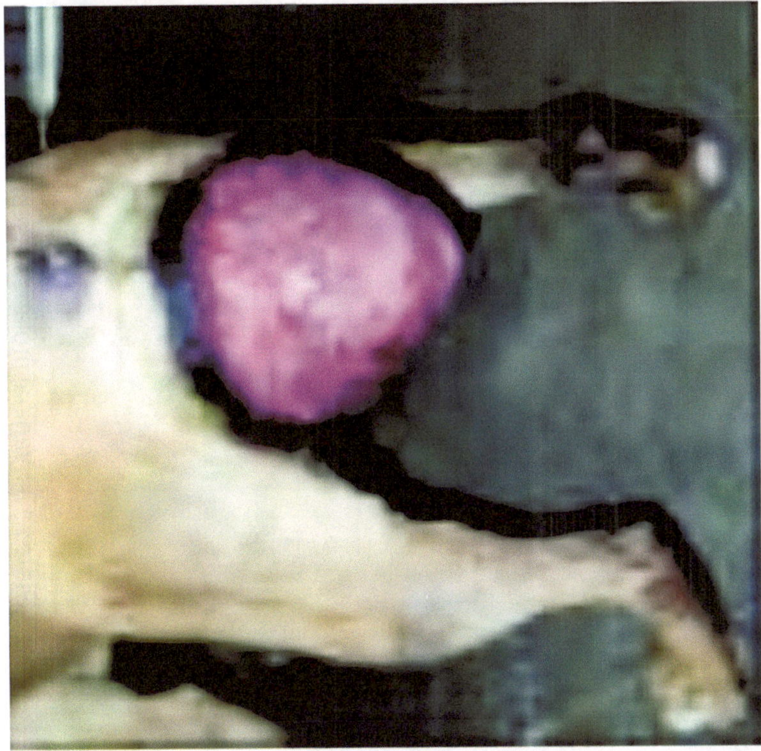

Plate - 12 : Vaginal prolapse in a bitch

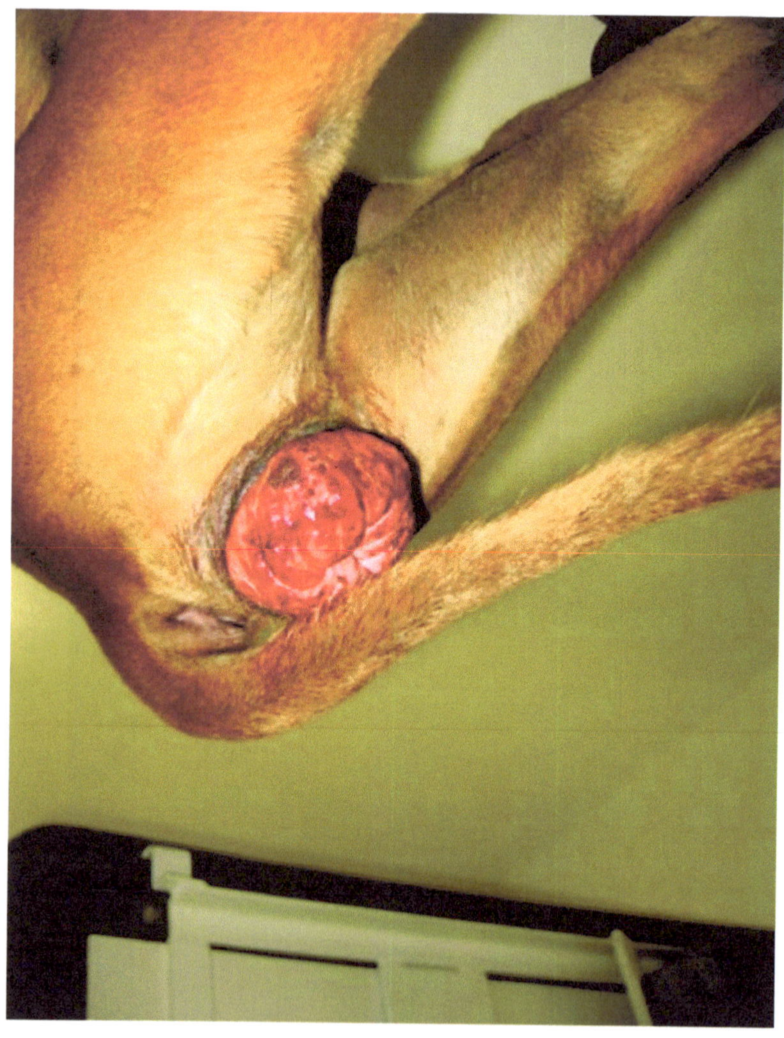

Plate - 13 : Vaginal prolapse in a bitch

Case-10

INFERTILITY IN BITCHES ASSOCIATED WITH UNDER SUPPLEMENTATION

- Various dietary deficiencies cause reproductive disorders.
- Protein deficiency causes delayed exhibition of first estrus, prolonged anestrus with agalactia.
- Essential fatty acids deficiency causes poor growth, fatty liver, degeneration of vital organs etc.
- Vit A affects degeneration and keratinization of epithelial cells of vagina and ovaries. Vit D retarded bone development. Deficiency of Vit E causes degeneration of germinal epithelium, failure of gestation and unusual estrous cycles.
- Mineral and trace elements deficiencies cause delayed puberty, prolonged anestrus and retarded growth.

Treatment

- Advice good balanced diet which contains all ingredients like; protein, minerals & vitamins as well as low fat and high fiber.
- Deworming the animal at regular intervals.
- Supplementation of feed with probiotics & vit E
- Feed the branded food like Fortiflora (Nestle), Purina (Petcare), VM 365 Tab (Intervet) etc.

Table 1 : Recommended nutrient allowance (% or amount / kg on dry matter basis) for an adult bitch

Nutrients	Bitch
Protein %	20
Linoleic acid %	1
Phosphorus %	0.9
Sodium %	1
Iron mg/kg	50
Vitamin A IU	5000
Vitamin E IU	60
Vitamin B_2 mg	2
Biotin mg	0.05
Fat %	5
Calcium %	1.2
Potassium %	0.5
Magnesium %	0.04
Zinc mg/kg	50
Vitamin D IU	400
Vitamin B_1 mg	1
Niacin mg	10
Choline mg	1000

Feeding schedule for female dogs

At 3 weeks	-	Good, small piece of meat, egg may be given.
3 weeks to 3 months	-	4-5 times feeding/ day
3 to 5 months	-	3 times a day
5 to 10 months	-	2 times a day
Adult	-	twice a day for maintenance
Lactating Female	-	Increased energy, protein etc.
Old female dogs	-	Improve the quality of feed, decreased the quantity.

Table 2: Example of home made foods for female dogs

Diet	**Body weight**	
	20 kg	**30 kg**
Milk (ml)	150	250
Fish (g)	50	50
Beef (g)	100-150	250-300
Rice (g)	100	150
Green vegetables	Ad lib (seasonal)	Ad lib (seasonal)
Vitamins (A+B+D etc.)	+	+
Bone meal	+	+
Salt	+	+

❑❑❑

Case-11

REPRODUCTIVE DISORDERS ASSOCIATED WITH OVER SUPPLEMENTATION IN BITCHES

- Obesity is indicated by 15% or more over ideal body weight.
- It leads to prolonged anestrus, infertility, weak uterine tone and lactational problems.

Causes

- Inappropriate diet
- Lack of exercise
- Genetic predisposition
- Hormonal disturbances

Treatment

- Follow weight control guidelines
- Increase exercise
- Reduce the amount of current diet and allow balanced diet or shift to low calorie diet (low fat & high fibre).

Case-12

PREGNANCY DIAGNOSIS IN BITCHES

- The ovaries of the bitch are necessary for the maintenance of pregnancy.
- In first 5 weeks of gestation, there is no increase in body weight but later on it is there.

Clinical Methods of PD

(A) Mammary glands

- At day 35, the teats become pink, enlarged, turgid, softer and tumified. On day 45 there is hypertrophy of mammary glands.

(B) Abdominal Palpation

- Depends on size of animals, temperament
- Period of gestation
- Number of fetuses in uteri
- Normal size or fatty bitch

i. Days 18-21:

   Fetus 12 mm long and 9 mm broad

ii. Days 24-30:

   Optimum period for PD, palpate conceptual swellings

iii. Days 35-44 and Day 45-55:

   Fast development

iv. Days 55-63: By manipulation of the abdomen

OR

Digital examination per rectum.

(C) Radiography

Fetal skeleton at 45 days onward.

(D) Ultrasonography

By Doppler method, real time by external transducer fetal heart sounds can be seen at 29th day.

(E) Laboratory Methods

i. By measurement of serum proteins: i.e; 3 fold rise in serum fibrinogen concentration at 4-5 weeks of mating.

ii. Rise in serum C-reactive protein (CRP)-Acute please proteins.

iii. Relaxin concentrations are elevated from 20-30 days of gestation but absent in nonpregnant at all stages.

❑❑❑

Case-13

METHODS OF POPULATION CONTROL IN BITCHES

There is no one best method of estrus (heat) control; the choice will vary for each animal. Spaying is irreversible and therefore, a safe and reversible alternative is needed.

Administration of Pharmaceutical Agents

1. Progesterone

(a) MAG (Magestrol acetate)

- Orally active progestagen
- Short half life (8days) in dogs
- Used for prevention & post ponement of estrus

Dose : Daily for 8 days at a dose of 2.2 mg/kg body wt.

(b) Delvosteron

- It provides a safe and reversible alternative
- Contains a second generation progestagen, proligestone and has several advantages, regarding safety, over other preparations.
- It can be used in different ways: Temporary as well as prolonged postponement of heat, suppression of heatetc.

2. Androgen

(a) Testosterone

- 25 mg orally weekly to keep out away from estrus for as longer 5 yrs.

(b) Mibolerone

- A synthetic 19- norsteroid compound is used for long term estrus inhibition.

  Dose: 30 mg/day to 12 kg body wt treated for a period of 1300 days.
- It is an androgenic, anabolic, anti gonadotropic steroid.

contd.....

Various Hormones Preparations used in Veterinary Gynaecology & Obstetrics

S.No.	Hormone	Preparation	Company Name
1	Proluton Depot	500mg / 2ml amp. 250mg / 1ml amp.	German Remedies
2	Duraprogen	250 mg/1ml amp. 500 mg/2ml amp. 750 mg/3ml amp.	Unichem
3	Uniprogestin	250 mg & 500 mg/ml (1&2 ml ampoule)	Foreva
4	Vetaprogen	250 mg/ml (2 ml ampoule)	Prima vetcare
5	Receptal (Gn RH analogue)	Buseraline acetate 4 µg/ml (10 ml & 2.5 ml vial)	Intervet
6	Gynarich (Gn RH analogue)	Buseraline acetate 4 µg/ml (2.5 ml & 5 ml vials)	Intas Pharmaceuticals Ltd.
7	Pragma	Each ml contains 250 µg cloprostenol (2 ml vial)	Intas Pharmaceuticals Ltd.
8	Lutalyse	25 mg/5 ml vial (5 mg Dinoporst prothamine per ml)	Pfizer
9	Cyclix	2 ml & 20 ml Vial Each ml contains 250 µg cloprostenol	Intervet
10	Prosolvin	7.5 mg/ml (2ml, 10ml vial)	Intervet

contd.....

11	Iliren	0.196 mg / ml (10 ml vial)	Intervet
12	Vetmate (PGF_2 alpha analogue)	2 ml Vial Each ml contains 250 μg cloprostenol	Vetcare
13	Folligon	1000 i.u. PMSG (each vial)	Intervet
14	Chorulon	1500 i.u. hCG (each vial)	Intervet
15	Norgestomet ear implant (CRESTAR)	3 mg norgestomet (ear imlant) 2ml inj (3mg norgestomet & 5 mg Estradiol valerate)	Intervet
16	Progynon	1 ml / ampoule (estradiol valerate 10 mg)	German Remedies
17	Vet Pitocin	5 I.U./0.5 ml (1 ml amp)	Parke-Davis
18	Syntocinon	5 I.U./ml (1 ml amp.)	Navartis

❑❑❑

Suggested Further Reading

1. Noakes, D.E., Parkinson, T.J. and England, G.C.W. (2009). Veterinary Reproduction and Obstetrics, 9th Edition, Saunders Publishers.

2. Tomar, N.S. (1976). Artificial Insemination and Reproduction of Cattle and Buffaloes, CSA University of Agriculture and Technology, Kanpur.

3. Mahmood, S. (2008). Instructional Manual on Systemic Approach to Artificial Insemination in bovines, Published by IVRI, Izatnagar, U.P.

4. Agarwal, S.K. and Tomar, O.S. (2003). Reproduction in Buffaloes, Published by IVRI, Izatnagar, U.P.

5. Kumar, H. (2004). Manual on Veterinary Obstetrics, Published by IVRI, Izatnagar, U.P.

6. Kumar, H. and Kumar, S. (2004). Pashu Prajanan evam Banjhpan : Samasyayen, Prabandhan evam Nidan, Published by IVRI, Izatnagar, U.P.

❏❏❏

About the Authors

Dr. Harendra Kumar born on 15th June, 1960. He completed his B.Sc., B.V.Sc. & A.H., M.V.Sc. and Ph.D. in Veterinary Gynaecology and Obstetrics. He has rich experience of more than 24 years in different capacities as Veterinary Assistant Surgeon, Scientist, Senior Scientist, Principal Scientist in the Division of Animal Reproduction, I.V.R.I., Izatnagar. He has guided 8 M.V.Sc. and Ph.D. students and about 100 research publications of national and international repute and more than 80 technical/popular articles. He has completed 12 research projects on various aspects of animal reproduction as P.I. He has attended more than 25 conferences and seminars. He is the recipient of Young Scientist Award, Prof. Neils Lagerlof Award by ISSAR and fellow of NAVS. He has written 2 technical bulletins, 1 manual and 1 book on animal reproduction. He has gained vast experience during handling the clinical cases at organized dairy farms, IVRI Polyclinics as well as in fields at farmer's door.

Dr. Sukdeb Nandi graduated in Veterinary Science and Animal Husbandry in 1986 from Bidhan Chandra Krishi Viswavidyalaya, Mohanpur, Nadia, W.B. He did his Master Degree and Ph.D. in Veterinary Virology from Deemed University, Indian Veterinary Research Institute in 1988 and 1992 respectively. He is also involved in imparting trainings on serological and molecular diagnosis of different Viral Diseases of animals. He was awarded with DBT sponsored National Biotechnology Associateship and carried out research on biotechnological and molecular techniques of diagnosing the diseases at Indian Institute of Chemical Biology, CSIR Institute at Jadavpur, Kolkata from 1995 to 1996. He was also deputed to United Kingdom in 1998-1999 to undergo 'Transfer of Molecular Biology Training' (TOMBIT) at Institute for Animal Health, Pirbight to work on molecular aspects of Foot and Mouth Disease Virus. He has carried out research on Rabies, FMD, Sheep Pox, Goat Pox, Bluetongue, Infectious Bovine Rhinotracheitis and Canine Parvovirus infections in canines. He has traveled different places in United Kingdom, Scotland and France, Presently, he is working as Senior Scientist at Centre for Animal Disease Research and Diagnosis, Indian Veterinary Research Institute, Izatnagar, U.P. He is also the author of 'Manual of Viral Disease Investigation' - a book very much useful for the scientists, teachers, students, diagnosticians and others who are working in this area. Other books in his credit are Veterinary Virology : at a glance, Immunology - at a glance, Animal Cell Culture and Virology, Avian influenza or Birdflu, Rabies : a killer disease, Veterinary Public Health - at a glance and Poultry Diseases - at a glance.

Dr. R.B. Rai, born on Jan. 5, 1954, completed his B.V.Sc. & AH, M.V.Sc. and Ph.D. in Veterinary Pathology from G.B. Pant U.A.&T, Pantnagar. He joined ARS in Sept. 1983 and served in CSWRI (Garsa, Kullu), CARI Port Blair and since Aug 2006 posted as Principal Scientist in IVRI. He served as Director, Animal Husbandry & Veterinary, services in A&D Islands with additional charges of Agriculture and Fisheries departments and Director, CARI, Port Blair.

He is recipient of many national awards including 'K.S. Nair Memorial Medal', ICAR Team Research Award (twice), 'Fakharuddin Ali Ahmad Award' (twice) and is fellow of National Academy of Agricultural Sciences, National Academy of Veterinary Science. He has published 180 research papers in national and international journals, 27 books (inlcuding 15 e-books) and delivered more than 170 lead/invited/contributory papers in National Seminars/Symposia.